A LOVED ONE WITH DEMENTIA

EMPOWERING YOU

The Rowman & Littlefield Empowering You series is aimed to help you, as a young adult, deal with important topics that you, your friends, or family might be facing. Whether you are looking for answers about certain illnesses, social issues, or personal problems, the books in this series provide you with the most up-to-date information. Throughout each book you will also find stories from other teenagers to provide personal perspectives on the subject.

A LOVED ONE WITH DEMENTIA

Insights and Tips for Teenagers

JEAN RAWITT

ROWMAN & LITTLEFIELD
Lanham • Boulder • New York • London

Published by Rowman & Littlefield
An imprint of The Rowman & Littlefield Publishing Group, Inc.
4501 Forbes Boulevard, Suite 200, Lanham, Maryland 20706
www.rowman.com

6 Tinworth Street, London, SE11 5AL, United Kingdom

British Library Cataloguing in Publication Information Available

Library of Congress Cataloging-in-Publication Data

Names: Rawitt, Jean, 1952– author.
Title: A loved one with dementia : insights and tips for teenagers / Jean
  Rawitt.
Description: Lanham : Rowman & Littlefield, [2021] | Series: Empowering you |
  Includes bibliographical references and index. | Summary: "This book
  addresses the challenges teenagers may face when a family member has
  dementia. It offers valuable information and support, with stories from
  young adults themselves and interviews with adults who know and care for
  people with dementia"— Provided by publisher.
Identifiers: LCCN 2020029322 (print) | LCCN 2020029323 (ebook) | ISBN
  9781538136980 (paperback) | ISBN 9781538136997 (ebook)
Subjects: LCSH: Dementia—Patients—Family relationships. |
  Dementia—Patients—Care. | Parent and teenager.
Classification: LCC RC521 .R39 2020 (print) | LCC RC521 (ebook) | DDC
  616.8/31—dc23
LC record available at https://lccn.loc.gov/2020029322
LC ebook record available at https://lccn.loc.gov/2020029323

CONTENTS

YOU ARE NOT ALONE

What is dementia? Let's start at the beginning. "Dementia is a disorder in which mental functions break down. It grows worse with time. It features personality change, confusion, and lack of energy. Thinking, reason, memory, and judgment are affected."[1] "Dementia is a nonreversible decline in mental function."[2] "Worldwide, around 50 million people have dementia. . . . Every year, there are nearly 10 million new cases. . . . The total number of people with dementia is projected to reach 82 million in 2030 and 152 in 2050."[3]

These facts explain very simply the definition and statistics that make dementia an important subject to be aware of. But why a book about dementia for teenagers?

First, because with more people marrying and having children later in life than in previous generations, and with the advances in medical care and general health allowing people to live longer lives, it is more likely than ever that young people will find themselves in close relationships with people who have dementia.

Second, because there is an important role teens can take in helping to improve the lives of people with dementia. This plays out not only in the direct contact teens may have with people experiencing cognitive decline, but also how the *world* deals with people with dementia and how teens can help shape that in a positive way.

Dementia can be a frightening and overwhelming disease, both for the person who is traveling through the downward stages of its path and their family, friends, and community. Because many people do not understand what dementia is and why and how it affects a person, it often causes embarrassment, stigmatization, or mistreatment. It can be so distressing that it causes people to become withdrawn from social contacts and can leave friends and relatives uncertain about how to behave with their loved one who has the disease or reluctant to acknowledge or accept the realities of the deterioration it can cause.

There are many ways in which you can create or continue to have a meaningful, beneficial, and even joyful relationship with someone who has dementia. Even though there is currently no cure, and even knowing that dementia is a terminal illness, you can develop and maintain a loving and positive interaction that can be deeply fulfilling and leave you with a feeling of gratification for having given of yourself to someone who truly needs that gift.

I was lucky to have two adoring and adored grandparents. They both lived into their late 90s, and until nearly the very end of their lives, they lived in an apartment together just blocks from where I lived with my parents and brothers. The Grands, as we called them, were our babysitters when we were young, and when we were too old to need babysitting, they were still very much active in our lives.

As we all got older, the tables turned, and they were the ones needing care. When I learned to drive, I helped by taking them grocery shopping. Little by little, they needed more and more help with things, and I loved to do what I could to help them. But by the time Grampa was in his late 90s, it was clear that he was confused and behaving in very disruptive ways, and my Gramma could no longer take care of him in their apartment. With our help, they moved to a nursing home, and we all hoped they'd make a good adjustment.

That was not to be the case. Grampa went into a downward spiral and died only a few days later. Gramma lived another year, at first making a few friends and enjoying some activities. But one night, waking up confused, she tried to get out of bed, fell, and broke her hip, and even though she had surgery to repair it, she never recovered.

I loved them. They lived good and long lives, but the ending was sad. Looking back, my mother and I realized not only how confused and disoriented Grampa had become, but also how Gramma, even though she managed to cover up a lot, had also deteriorated mentally over the last few years. We felt that we should have realized that sooner, and if we had, perhaps we could have done something that would have helped.

Our story is not unusual, but the impact it made on me was life-changing. By the time my grandparents died, I was already well along in a career I loved. One of my colleagues was an elderly gentleman who had already retired once, only to return to his old office to take on small projects and mentor the younger staff and share his expertise. I adored him, learned from him, and enjoyed his company enormously. But one day he suffered a stroke at work, and then he, too, began to experience a cognitive decline (decline in his mental skills). I visited him often, but it was sad to watch him lose his abilities in small increments.

Not long after his death, I decided to step away from my career. With time on my hands, I applied to become a volunteer at my local hospital. When the director of volunteers asked where I would like to work, I answered, "I'd like to work with geriatric patients." Her answer came quickly: "Wonderful! No one wants to work with older patients!" And so began a second career.

Since that time, I have always been involved, in some way, in the care of the old. Some have been my own family, some have been my friends, and some have been strangers who became dear friends. Taking care of them, being involved in their lives as they grew frail, lost their physical abilities, and, in many cases, lost their cognitive ability, their ability to think, remember, and even recognize me or know who they were themselves, has been an emotionally draining but enormously gratifying part of my life. In some ways, it is terrifying—because I know, from close and intimate experience, what might happen. But I have also learned that the best way to face the fear is to learn as much as I can about whatever it is that scares me. With dementia, I knew that I needed to learn as much as I could about it and then let myself experience the difficult emotional roller coaster that loving someone with diminishing cognition becomes. Throughout this time, however, I knew that I was deeply grateful to be able to bring joy, attention, and love to these people, even when they no longer knew who I was. They made my life infinitely richer and more meaningful, and were always a source of creativity and inspiration.

Our population is growing older, and people are living much longer than they used to. Many people are starting families later, so that their children are growing up with older grandparents, as well as older parents. While advances in medicine have, in many ways, enabled people to live longer and healthier lives, a growing number of people will experience some form of dementia in their later years.

While there are no cures at this time for most, if not all, forms of dementia, there are many things we can do to help people deal with its effects, understand how best to confront it, and be generous and useful to those who experience it. We can learn ways to entertain those whose minds are no longer able to process information as they used to. We can discover ways to soothe and comfort the frustrations, anxieties, and even anger of those whose minds are slipping. There are physical things we can do, ways we can learn to communicate better, and ways to interact more effectively with those who have lost the abilities they once had. And we can find ways to help those who feel they have lost their sense of purpose and usefulness, which is so necessary to making life worthwhile.

Al, a young man who watched his grandmother's years-long decline from Alzheimer's disease, put it simply: "It's great to have things to do, great to have ways to provide comfort. But because there's nothing you can fix, you can just really *be* there. That's all they really want."

Dealing with someone who has dementia—no matter how much you care about them—can be very difficult and affect you in many ways. Because it is a disease that profoundly changes the person you know, changing their behaviors, moods, memory, physical abilities, and abilities to care for themselves, it can cause many mixed emotions in the people who care about them. It can—very often at the same time—create feelings of confusion, guilt, avoidance, and frustration, as well as acceptance, compassion, and deepening love. Caring for someone with dementia can require a bottomless pool of patience and strength, but it can be a source of equally deep gratification. It can be a time that requires a great deal from you, but because of the nature of the illness, we know that it will have a definite end point.

Having a family member with dementia also profoundly affects the family dynamic. The stress of caring for their parent can cause *your* parent to be on edge, short-tempered, and even depressed. It can cause strain on a marriage; it can put the burden of extra tasks and responsibilities on family members—not only the immediate family, but also the extended family. It can cause financial burdens, and it can cause feelings of guilt. Knowing how this disease can affect an entire family and thinking about it and learning ways to respond in helpful rather than negative ways can help ease some of the tension.

Even more basic than the practical things teenagers can do when dealing with someone with dementia, there is one important point to keep in mind: For many, if not most, older people—whether cognitively intact or in cognitive decline—seeing a bright, cheerful, young face, whether that of a dear family member or a yet-to-be-known friend, lifts their mood. Having a young person visit, whether engaging in conversation or an activity, or just sitting with them—being "in the moment" with them—has the power to ease loneliness, lighten a depressed mood, distract them from pain or sadness, and *bring them back* into the world they may feel they are leaving or have left. This is a huge gift that you can bring. It can be almost magical, and it requires no tools, no special knowledge, no experience, just willingness and a smile.

Most importantly, by understanding more about the illness and our feelings about it, and learning what we can do to help, we can be better prepared to handle and empathize with the changes our loved ones experience as they journey along the path of cognitive decline. Even more, we can learn to appreciate them for who they are, and who they continue to be, despite the changes we see. As Carey Mulligan, actress and spokesperson for the Alzheimer's Society, reminds us, "Those with dementia are still people, and they still have stories and they still have character, and they're all individuals and they're all unique. And they just need to be interacted with on a human level."[4]

Young people have the power to positively impact the lives of individuals with dementia, as well as help others understand why that is both possible and important to do. Teens can be ambassadors to that unfamiliar territory; they can help destigmatize the disease, advocate for those with the disease, and help change the way their friends, their community, and even the greater society look at and deal with people with dementia. So, my message to you is, learn all you can, open your heart, and bring light to those who are facing the darkening world ahead.

NOTE TO THE READER

Throughout this book, I have chosen to illustrate suggestions or anecdotes by writing about "your grandmother" or "your grandfather." I recognize that the person with dementia in your life may not be a grandparent or even a relative. They may be a family friend, a neighbor, or someone with whom you work or for whom you volunteer. To keep things simple and straightforward, I have chosen to refer to that person most often as your grandparent. Consider it an homage to my own Grands.

To the many adults and professionals who offered their stories, wisdom, knowledge, and expertise, thank you for your support and information. To the many young people who opened up to me about their experiences loving or caring for someone with dementia, thank you, thank you. Your honesty and generosity in talking with me about your feelings, concerns, fears, and questions helped shape this book and—I hope—give life and color to a very tough subject.

PART I

WHAT IS DEMENTIA?

CHAPTER ONE

WHAT IS DEMENTIA?

Dementia is the loss of cognitive functioning—thinking, remembering, and reasoning—and behavioral abilities to such an extent that it interferes with a person's daily life and activities. These functions include memory, language skills, visual perception, problem-solving, self-management, and the ability to focus and pay attention. Some people with dementia cannot control their emotions, and their personalities may change. Dementia ranges in severity from the mildest stage, when it is just beginning to affect a person's functioning, to the most severe stage, when the person must depend completely on others for basic activities of living.[1]

Sir Terry Pratchett, world-renowned author of the Discworld series, wrote of his own experience with dementia: "It's a nasty disease, surrounded by shadows and small, largely unseen tragedies. People don't know what to say unless they have it in the family."[2]

Some people describe the changes in memory that take place in dementia as being like Swiss cheese, with different-sized holes perforating the memory like the holes in the cheese. Others liken it to a chalkboard, in which whatever is written on the board continually gets erased from the bottom up. Whatever the picturesque description used to describe the memory loss of dementia, there is no question that it is devastating and has an impact on every aspect of daily life.

What dementia is *not*, is a normal part of aging. Although, as people age, muscles grow weaker, bones may become more brittle, and people tend to slow down, they do not necessarily fall victim to the progressive cognitive losses of dementia. They may think or process information more slowly than when they were younger, and they may occasionally forget things, but for many people, while those issues might be frustrations of daily life, they do not signal the more profound, inexorable, and debilitating onset of dementia. The most significant factor in the difference between the changes of normal aging and symptoms of a disease is when the cognitive issues interfere with a person's ability to function in daily life.

Most cases of dementia are diagnosed after age sixty-five; however, it is not solely a disease of old age. Some two hundred thousand cases of dementia per year occur in people in their 40s or 50s; these are generally considered cases of early-onset dementia. Therefore, while it can occur in middle-aged people, most cases are seen in people of more advanced age.

Although Alzheimer's disease may be what most people think of when they think of dementia, as it accounts for about 60 to 70 percent of cases, there are other forms of dementia. In addition to Alzheimer's disease, these include vascular dementia, Lewy body dementia, and fronto-temporal dementia it is possible for someone to have more than one of these at the same time. The causes and symptoms of these forms of dementia are somewhat different, but symptoms can include, in addition to memory loss, changes in personality and behavior, losses in language, confusion, and changes in sleep patterns. People may also experience dementia as a result of a side effect of medication, a vitamin deficiency, or a thyroid condition; luckily, these forms of dementia are generally reversible if treated appropriately.[3] Drinking too much alcohol; suffering a head injury; or even emotional issues such as stress, anxiety, or depression can cause memory problems that look like dementia but clear up if the issues are treated.[4]

True dementia, however, is not yet curable. While there are some treatments that have been shown to help slow the progress of the disease in some people and there are some medications that can help ease some of the symptoms, at this time there is no known cure. Scientists throughout the world are working on many different approaches to finding a cure because dementia is a devastating problem worldwide. Some exciting areas of research that scientists are working on include developing new drugs that may target the causes of dementia, exploring the impact of inflammation on the development of dementia, and studying how dietary or caloric restriction may serve as a way to either prevent or slow the course of the disease.

While finding ways to prevent, slow, or cure the progress of Alzheimer's disease and other forms of dementia is tremendously important, until ways to do that are found, it is also vital to find better ways to care for people with dementia on a daily basis. Much research is being done to find ways to improve the quality of life for people with dementia, including in such areas as environmental design, personal care, individual decision-making, how certain words and language can impact feelings of isolation and stigma for people with dementia, and even how virtual reality can be used to help improve the quality of life for people with advanced dementia.

OPPORTUNITIES TO PARTICIPATE IN RESEARCH

The National Institute on Aging supports research at major medical institutions through the Alzheimer's Disease Research Centers (ADRCs). Scientists at the ADRCs are working on finding a way to cure—or even prevent—Alzheimer's disease, as well as ways to improve diagnosis and care for people with Alzheimer's disease. There are opportunities through the ADRCs for people—both healthy individuals and people with symptoms of the disease—to participate in research studies. In addition, there are support groups for patients and families.[5] The National Institute on Aging provides information on the ADRCs nearest to where you live and links to helpful resources (https://www .nia.nih.gov/health/alzheimers-disease-research-centers).

HATTIE'S STORY: HOW A YOUNG WOMAN BECAME INVOLVED IN DEMENTIA RESEARCH

Hattie has always been drawn to community service, volunteering through school programs even as a young girl. When she was in middle school, she joined an after-school program called Sweet Readers, which trains middle-school students to engage with older people with dementia in art projects as a way to enhance and expand intergenerational connections and understanding. After participating in the Sweet Readers program for a year, Hattie decided she wanted to continue working with people with dementia and volunteered at a neighborhood senior center that had a daycare program for people with moderate to severe dementia.

"I had never been with people who were nonverbal or who could no longer move, so that was a whole other level of interaction for me, and I found it tremendously rewarding," Hattie said.

> And, later in the summer, I started doing my research into Alzheimer's disease and dementia—reading scientific articles and whatever I could find to understand the disease more. When I had the opportunity to attend a two-week summer program in Cambridge, England, I ended up turning my interest into a presentation project for my course in social psychology. At first, I was going to do a project on the aging population, but then I decided just to change it to dementia because I wanted to focus more specifically on that.
>
> After that program finished, I realized I wanted to learn even more about dementia. Since then, I've been researching on the weekends, and I'm now working on a website where I want to post articles, write a blog, and inform people about the disease. It's a huge challenge, but I feel that there's so much I want people to know, especially about how isolating the disease is and how things can improve for people with dementia.

I still have to finish high school, but I know I want to go into a field like neuroscience, or geriatrics, or some other area of science where I can expand this interest. For now, I'm just reading all I can about it.

There are also indications that certain lifestyle changes can help prevent the onset of diseases like Alzheimer's. The benefits of increasing physical activity, reducing hypertension (high blood pressure), and engaging in cognitive training (brain exercises) as a preventative against dementia are exciting and promising areas of research, as well as ways in which individuals can take some control over their continuing health.[6]

A PROFESSIONAL'S ADVICE: LEARNING ABOUT THE DISEASE WILL HELP YOU COPE WITH IT

Grace, a social worker who works with people with dementia and their families, often meets with families who are dealing with dementia. Her perspective was sensible and straightforward.

The more you know, the better able you will be to deal with the effects of the disease. There can be so much frustration and anger, and a tendency to take things personally when you don't understand the disease. When you aren't familiar with it, you might think that the person with dementia is acting out or saying things to spite you, that they're doing it to make you mad. But if you learn a little bit about what's happening in the brain of someone with dementia, you realize that their social restraints may be lost, and their coping strategies are not there anymore. If you're able to think about putting yourself in their shoes and can ask yourself, for example, "How would I react if someone I didn't recognize walked into my house and tried to take off my clothes?" you begin to realize what it might be like and why you'd lash out, or yell, or struggle. But it's possible to learn how you can better approach someone, to learn a calming approach, how it's important to always introduce yourself, that it can be valuable to talk about the past, things that someone was interested in, whatever reaches them still; these are things you can learn that will help you both. You will find that even through the fog of dementia, you can find a way to connect that's meaningful and rewarding.

According to the World Health Organization, nearly 50 million people throughout the world have dementia, and there are almost 10 million new cases each year. The proportion of people age sixty and older living with dementia is 5 to 8 percent of the global population. It is estimated that the total number of people with dementia worldwide will reach 82 million by 2030, and 152 million by 2050.[7] The financial costs are tremendous, and the emotional and social toll is unmeasurable. Dementia, therefore, presents an enormous burden not only on the individual with dementia, but also on their families, caregivers, and communities—and on the entire global health system.

CHAPTER TWO

WHAT DOES DEMENTIA LOOK LIKE?

Whatever happens, you know that it's going to be like a very bumpy ride.
—Josef, a young man who watched his grandmother die of dementia

Dementia is usually—although not always—noticeable. Some people with dementia, especially in the early stages, look and act as they always did, and may deal with the symptoms with casual acceptance. Many people can cover up their deficits with good social skills or habits retained from long ago. For example, it is said that Ralph Waldo Emerson, noted author, essayist, and leader of the American Transcendentalist movement in the mid-nineteenth century, who suffered from mental decline in his later years, would answer, when asked about his health, "I have lost my mental faculties, but am perfectly well." For some people, dementia begins to become evident in innocuous ways, for example, in seeming to be unusually worried about the time or the weather; these concerns may appear to be an unusual quirk or habit they've developed.

As the disease progresses, it may become more obvious that your grandmother seems to forget what she is doing, or can't think of a word, or asks a question that doesn't seem to make sense or is not relevant to the conversation. Over time, in general, a person who has dementia will begin to look somewhat lost, as though they don't know where they are or who you are. One young man, Jonathan, when describing his grandmother at that stage, remembers her as seeming "disengaged." They may occasionally appear frightened or agitated. Their grooming habits may begin to erode; they may start to look unkempt, forgetting to comb or brush their hair, or shave; their clothing may begin to look worn, or stained, or unchanged for days. Their movements may become fidgety; they may wander around as if they don't know where they are or where they are going.

Khadija, a young woman who volunteers with dementia patients at a nursing home, described what she sees as follows: "Since I've been coming here, I've gotten used to seeing the progression. There are residents I first saw two years ago who seemed in great health. But since then, as I've seen them over time, it's as though slowly, they're losing bits and pieces of themselves."

When the disease progresses into the late stages, your grandparent may no longer be able to stand without help, sit upright in a chair, or feed themselves. While every individual is different, there are relatively predictable stages and manifestations to the progress of dementia, although there is no set schedule as to how long these stages go on; indeed, it is often unclear when a person has passed from one stage to another. As the course of the disease develops, the issues and difficulties will increase, and life—for the individual with dementia and their family and caregivers—will become more complicated. As Josef, a young man who watched his grandmother die of dementia and now works as a volunteer with patients in the memory care unit of a nursing home, said, "Whatever happens, you know that it's going to be like a very bumpy ride."

EARLY COGNITIVE DECLINE/ EARLY-STAGE DEMENTIA

In the earliest stages, you might not notice that anything is different about your grandmother, except that she always seems to be worried about what time it is or whether you can get home before dark. In the earliest stages, dementia can cause lapses in short-term memory, the most recent memories; for example, you might ask your grandmother what she had for breakfast and find her answering, "I think I had eggs, yes, I had eggs. And probably toast. Or maybe it was cereal." In other ways, she may be going about her daily business as she always has. She may socialize with friends, prepare meals, and shop—but you may begin to hear about problems that arise as she does. She may mention that her friends accused her of forgetting the cards she played in their weekly bridge game or laugh that she served mashed potatoes and string beans for dinner but forgot to cook the meat she had bought. Simple daily experiences that never gave her trouble before may begin to cause her problems.

ERICA'S DAD: REALIZING SOMETHING IS WRONG

My dad is an old-school Italian. He's a very proud man, but he would often lose things or misplace things; it was just something he did. Then we started to see that he would always shift the blame; instead of saying, "I don't know where my keys are," he'd lash out angrily with, "Who moved my keys?" or "Why'd you move my keys?" He'd always find someone to blame instead of thinking it was something he'd done.

Then one day, he went out to go hunting with my brothers. That was always something they would do together; they would spend hours in the woods; they'd scout out places. On that day, I remember that they called home in the afternoon, and said, "Just so you know, Dad didn't meet us at the rendezvous point, we're not sure where he is, and we think he's lost in the woods." That was very bizarre for him; they used to hunt from the same spot all the time. Luckily, they found him, just after dark. But it was those kinds of things that keyed us in to realizing that something bigger was going on. We started to realize that this was not just Dad occasionally losing his keys.

So much of our daily life is dependent on our remembering things that we often don't realize what a problem it is when we no longer can: remembering a PIN to use the cash machine, remembering an appointment, remembering where we put our keys, remembering the way home, or remembering to turn off the stove. When being unable to remember these things is no longer an occasional occurrence but becomes a daily, and disturbing, issue, is when it becomes likely to be labeled dementia.

MID-STAGE/MODERATE DEMENTIA

In the middle stages, things begin to become more difficult and more noticeable. Your grandmother may not remember that she had breakfast—and eat breakfast again. She may forget to take her medications—or take them again. This stage is generally the one where it becomes clear that Grandmother will need some help to manage her day-to-day life. She may need someone to help for a few hours a day with personal care, perhaps setting up her medications, or help her shop or prepare her meals. It may become evident that she needs someone with her when she ventures outside her home because she has become lost in the neighborhood a few times or confused in her local store or bank, needing help from clerks or strangers. Your family may get a call from someone that they found your grandmother wandering in the neighborhood and unsure of how to get home; she may have even stopped someone and asked for help. Taking care of personal hygiene may become more complicated, as people become more forgetful and confused.

ERICA'S DAD: DAILY LIFE BECOMES MORE DIFFICULT

My dad is starting to wander more. It gets a little difficult at night. I know my mom's trying to find the most appropriate alarm system, something that would allow him to wander around the house—after all, you can't just lock someone in the bedroom—but keep him safe. My parents live on a main road, so if he wanders outside, it's terrifying to think what could happen.

The other thing is that even though he seems to be doing pretty well, he needs a lot of prompting about some things. Like, "Oh, Dad, you have to take a shower today." Then sometimes he'll take three showers in one day and not know what he's doing. He was doing okay most of the time, but then he had an episode of acting out, and they had to put him in the hospital because they thought he could be a danger to himself or other people. Since he came back from the hospital, it's been more of a struggle. He came back wearing adult diapers; he couldn't shower himself, or it took hours to shower him because he didn't understand any of the directions, and he was very lethargic. He's gotten a lot better recently, but he still needs help in the shower, or he'll go to the bathroom and then not know what to do, and my mom has to go help him.

MEDICATIONS

While there are some medications that can help alleviate some of the symptoms of dementia—there are medications that can help soothe anxiety, relieve paranoia, aid in sleep or wakefulness, and help modulate emotions—most have side effects that can be as troubling or hard to control as the symptoms they are intended to alleviate. Some medicines cause sleep disturbance, making a person either more wakeful or sleepier. Some medicines can cause someone to drool, a side effect that can be very distressing to the patient and challenging to handle. Some medications can cause dizziness and unstable balance or weakness, which can make walking or standing a safety issue. A careful and knowledgeable doctor will take into consideration all the medications a person takes and evaluate how they may react with one another, as well as what side effects they may cause. Sometimes, the decision about which drugs to prescribe will be a difficult one, as the doctor—and the family, if the individual is not able to make a decision—must weigh the benefits and risks of the effects the medications may have.

FALLS

One particular safety hazard at this stage is falling; whether because of medication interactions, physical weakness, or increased instability, a person with advancing dementia often suffers falls, whether indoors or on the street. They may try to explain it away by saying, "There was an uneven sidewalk, and I tripped," or, "I didn't see the curb," or, "I was trying to reach the shelf, and I fell," or even, "I don't know how I fell! One minute I was fine, and then I was on the ground." An increasing number of falls is usually a clue to advancing dementia.

POOR JUDGMENT AND SUSCEPTIBILITY TO FRAUD AND CRIME

Someone at this stage of dementia begins to show signs of poor judgment, such as trying to stand on a step stool (or worse, a chair) to reach something and losing their balance. They may try to heat their home by turning on the oven and leaving the oven open. My grandmother, in a particularly dangerous effort, couldn't reach a wall clock that had stopped working and used scissors to cut the electrical cord, which was still plugged in. Luckily, she suffered no injury, but it could have had a devastating effect. Sometimes poor judgment can lead to incidents that—in retrospect—can be hilarious but could have been tragic.

GRAMMA'S BIG ADVENTURE

When my mother (her grandchildren called her Gramma, as I had called *her* mother), was in the moderate stages of dementia, she was still able to ambulate with a walker but was never left alone because her judgment was poor. She lived in her apartment, across the street from where I live, and an aide was with her all the time. One evening, ten or twelve members of our family had gathered at my apartment, some from out of town. Although a few had visited Gramma individually earlier that day, we had decided not to bring my mother over, as we had noticed that being in a group of people, even when they were her own family, made her anxious and uncomfortable. Although she was, by that time, quite confused and unable to keep thoughts straight in her mind, she somehow sensed that her loved ones were "having a party" and decided she did not want to stay home. She managed to get herself out of her apartment when her helper's back was turned and had already gotten herself into the elevator and out of the lobby before the aide was able to follow.

Her aide immediately called me, crying, "Your mother got away from me and went downstairs!" I grabbed my keys and my brother, and we raced down to the street, only to be confronted by a huge, chanting, marching crowd of people parading down the avenue that separated our building from my mother's. It was a nightmarish scene—a political demonstration and rally, with placards, police cars, and hundreds of people blocking our way in the night, police lights flashing red and blue against the buildings.

We were frantic; it was almost impossible to cross the street, but we finally made it across, scanning the sidewalks, looking for a little old lady pushing a walker. My brother and I split up to search in opposite directions, terrified that my mother would wander far or even into the midst of the rally. We had just rejoined one another after a fruitless race around the block when my cell phone rang. It was my sister-in-law, calling from my apartment: "Mom's here."

Somehow, my frail, demented, walker-pushing ninety-two-year-old mother had made her way across the street, through the angry, chanting crowds, and upstairs to my apartment to join the party. When my brother and I made it back upstairs, breathless and drenched in a panicked sweat, we found Mom sitting calmly among her family, totally unfazed, never having noticed the chanting crowds, the police, or the nightmarish quality of the scene outside.

We were lucky; Mom was unharmed, undisturbed, and unaware of the danger in which she'd put herself. I, however, was wrung out by the terror I'd experienced when I thought we'd lost her and depleted by the recognition of how advanced her illness had become.

People at this stage are particularly vulnerable to fraud and deception. Scam artists are aware of this and often target older people they suspect may be easily fooled. They may convince them in a telephone call to wire money from their bank account to someone else, using a heartrending story to lure them into doing it. They may attempt—or succeed—to sell them fraudulent insurance policies or utility contracts, only benefiting themselves. Unscrupulous people may try to convince them to pay in advance for home repairs or household help and never deliver the services. It is not uncommon for thieves to watch a bank ATM vestibule for a vulnerable-looking older person, follow them in, engage them in a story about having been robbed or lost a wallet, and convince them to withdraw money to give them. A person who has cognitive impairments can be easily taken in not only because they don't recognize a fraudulent story, but also are no longer confident of their own abilities to detect a scam.

Similarly, people in early to mid-stage dementia are too often the victims of street crime. Activities that may not be difficult for a fully cognizant or younger person, such as getting off a bus while holding a package and a handbag, can be more difficult to coordinate for someone with cognitive deficits, and their slower way of moving leaves them ripe for a pickpocket to steal a wallet or a thief to grab a bag. They may move more slowly, have a look of confusion in their eyes, or appear uncertain—all of which makes them an easy mark for an unscrupulous person.

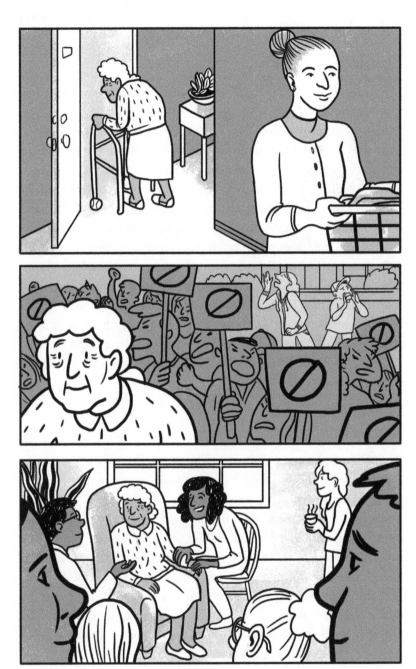

Sensing her family having a party across the street, Jean's mother got away from her aide and crossed the street, passing through the middle of a political rally, to reach her family on the other side. *Illustration by Kate Haberer*

"SUNDOWN SYNDROME"

Later-stage dementia also frequently causes the sense of time to become topsy-turvy. "Sundown syndrome," or "sundowning," is a common symptom for many people who have dementia. During the late afternoon and evening—the sundown hours—people often become more confused, more agitated, and more restless. They can become argumentative, angry, and frustrated. They might demand to go outside or refuse to bathe or eat—insisting that it is not bath time or dinnertime. The confusion and agitation caused by sundowning can be especially distressing for caregivers, as it can be very hard to reorient the individual's sense of time or dissuade them from their confused intentions. Oftentimes, if possible, it is best to go along with their version of reality, rather than try to persuade them otherwise. Alternatively, this is a time when finding a way to distract them may help, such as by trying to engage them in watching a TV show, playing a card game, or taking a walk. It can, however, be tough to penetrate the confusion of sundowning.

Getting Creative to Combat Sundowning

Because sundowning and disturbances in the sleep–wake cycle are a common symptom of dementia, many people show restlessness and increased activity in the late afternoon and evening hours, and sometimes even during the middle of the night. Sometimes encouraging more activity, like taking a longer evening walk, if possible, can help by tiring a person out, enabling them to sleep better during the night. If going outdoors is not an option, even pacing within the house can help. Find the longest hallway you can, and "take a walk" back and forth with them. Make it a game—"Let's see how many times we can touch the wall at either end!" Even better, turn on some music, and see if you can get some dance action going.

DIFFICULTIES WITH COMMUNICATION
AND EXPRESSIVENESS

As the disease progresses, a person with dementia may start to look a little blank when someone is speaking to them; you might note that their face looks expressionless, and it's as though they're not looking at anything or responding to what was said. Most likely, this is because either they are not able to understand what is being said or they don't recognize that someone is speaking to them. Indeed, sometimes a person with advancing dementia appears to deliberately "tune out" when the difficulty of trying to follow a conversation becomes overwhelming.

SOMETHING TO THINK ABOUT:
HEARING LOSS OR DEMENTIA?

While a person with dementia may seem not to understand what you're saying or not even know you are talking to them, keep in mind that there may be a reason *other* than the fact that they have dementia for this inattentiveness. They may be hard of hearing and not able to hear what you say.

Many older people suffer from hearing loss; sometimes, this is diagnosed and corrected with hearing aids. Sometimes people have hearing aids but don't use them; they may forget to put them in; they may find them uncomfortable or difficult to get used to; or they may forget, or be unable to put in batteries, or be unable to charge their rechargeable batteries. Moreover, hearing aids are generally very small and may be hard—particularly for someone with arthritis or some cognitive decline—to insert correctly or adjust or change the batteries because the controls are so tiny. So, while many people *have* hearing aids, many of them stop using them or use them incorrectly.

For many people, hearing aids are too expensive to get. The cost of hearing aids is generally not covered by medical insurance, and for that reason, many people who could benefit from them find them financially out of reach.

Someone can mistake the *inability to hear* for dementia. Very often someone who cannot hear a conversation will try to cover up that inability due to embarrassment or reluctance to admit they cannot hear. They may nod their head, look at the speaker, and *seem* to be participating in the conversation—until asked a question or to volunteer a comment, only to say something irrelevant to the actual discussion. When that happens, those around them may *assume* that they are demented—never considering that they may have just not heard what was said.

The ability to use words correctly, be able to retrieve appropriate words and use them effectively in a sentence, and engage in the interchange that is a conversation becomes harder and harder for a person with dementia. They may struggle to find a word, use a word *similar* to the one they intended, and even substitute a completely different word that does not make sense in the context of the conversation. Particularly for a person who enjoyed conversation, losing the ability to find words and put them together appropriately can be enormously frustrating and disheartening.

LOSS OF RECOGNITION OF FAMILIAR FACES

Khadija, a volunteer in a nursing home, knows that most of the time, the residents with whom she works do not remember her from week to week. "But some of the people, when I walk in, start blowing me kisses," she said.

> Some say, "I love you, I love you!" and I know they're happy to see me, even though I know they don't know my name and maybe don't know who I am. So it makes me wonder, do people remember feelings? Even if they don't know your face, or your name, or who you are, do they remember the way you made them feel, and when they see you again, do they feel that feeling again?

One of the hardest things to deal with is when someone you love or care about becomes so cognitively impaired—so demented—that they no longer recognize you. It is painful to have your beloved grandmother look right at you and not know your name or not remember that you are her grandchild; she might ask, "Do I know you?" or "Who are you?" She might even become upset or angry and tell you (or yell at you), "Get away! I don't know you!" She might imagine that you are someone else entirely: She might think that you are your parent when *they* were a child, or even see you as a stranger or someone scary.

This loss of recognition of familiar people can be tough to experience—for both of you. For you, it can be heartbreaking not to be recognized; for your grandmother, it can be frustrating and saddening. You can try, gently, to correct her: "It's me, Gramma, Susie, your granddaughter!" She may refuse to believe that and continue to insist that you are someone else. Usually, in that case, the best thing is to go along with her—agree with what she says or just accept it, and let her express whatever it is that works best for her. Trying to correct someone with dementia is rarely productive and often makes things worse.

ERICA'S DAD: FORGETTING FAMILIAR FACES

Lately, my dad is confused about who my mother is. He will often identify her by her name, Cathy, but he has trouble recognizing that she's his wife and my mother. At times, he thinks that I'm my mom and calls me by her name. A few months ago, he called my cell phone at 1 a.m., asking, "Where's your mother? She's been out all night," even though she was just in the other room. Even so, he still seems to have this sense that Mom is someone important to him, even though he doesn't seem to know who she is. He worries about her when she goes out, he follows her around, he's protective of her. But he just doesn't seem to know who she is."

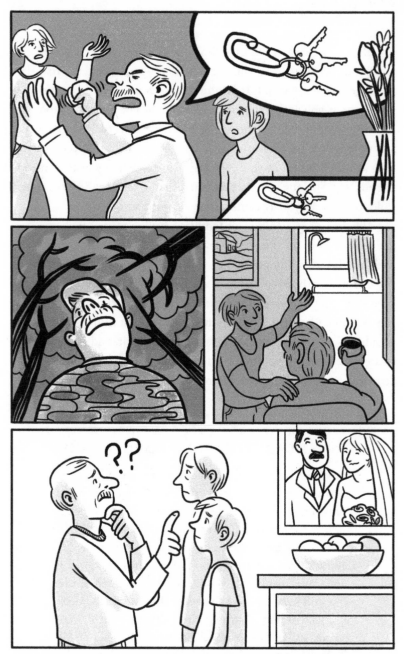

Erica's dad's dementia progressed from his misplacing things and forgetting tasks to wandering off and getting confused about important people in his life.
Illustration by Kate Haberer

LATER-STAGE DEMENTIA

If a person with advancing dementia has caring, thoughtful, and attentive help, they will generally be kept clean, fresh-smelling, clothed neatly and appropriately, and well-groomed. But, inevitably after a point, their eyes will begin to look blank, their faces will lose most expression, and their physical movement and behavior will be less under their control.

DECLINING APPETITE AND REDUCED INTAKE OF FOOD AND FLUIDS

One of the very difficult issues of later-stage dementia is nutrition (taking in foods) and hydration (taking in fluids). While the body requires sufficient nutrients and water to sustain it, as dementia progresses, both appetite and the ability to eat diminish. The sense of taste and smell—essential to the enjoyment of food—begin to be lost, even in normal aging. Chewing may become difficult, either because of dental problems or physical motor coordination. It may become necessary to puree food and hand-feed a person with advanced dementia to have them take in food. In late-stage dementia, a person begins to forget to swallow; this reflex, something we develop at the earliest point of our lives, is lost. For a while, this reflex can be encouraged by verbal reminders or even gentle stroking of the throat, but at a certain point, a person with end-stage dementia will begin to refuse food and drink. Even a person with severe dementia may clamp their lips shut or turn their head to prevent a spoon from being put in their mouth. Gentle and patient encouragement may prolong that period, but, ultimately, nutritional intake lessens and will eventually cease.

FRAILTY AND INCREASED RISK OF INFECTION

The frailer a person with dementia becomes, the weaker their immune system is and the more susceptible they are to infection. A scratch or tear in the skin, especially the skin breakdown known as a bedsore, can become a major and deadly infection. The inability to control urinary and bowel functions (incontinence) can lead to frequent urinary tract infections (UTIs). When a frail older person's immune system is not strong enough to fight them off, flu and pneumonia can quickly become fatal. The decision of how, or whether, to treat such infections can be an extremely difficult one to make; family caregivers and the doctor often must balance the consideration of "quality of life" against the complications—or downside—of treatment.

One particular danger, when the ability to swallow effectively begins to be lost, is that of developing what is called "aspiration pneumonia"—when food or liquid "goes down the wrong tube" and ends up in the lungs, causing an infection and pneumonia that can lead to death. Similarly, viral or bacterial pneumonia, sometimes called "community-acquired pneumonia," while usually treatable in healthy, younger people, can prove deadly to frail older people.

PNEUMONIA: "THE OLD MAN'S FRIEND"

Pneumonia has often been referred to as the "old man's friend," because it often occurs in frail, elderly people with weakened immune systems and who, when the pneumonia is left untreated, generally lapse into unconsciousness and die with little distress. Sir William Ostler, one of the founders of Johns Hopkins Hospital, who is often called the "Father of Modern Medicine," wrote in the first edition of his most famous work, *The Principles and Practice of Medicine* (1892), "In children and in healthy adults the outlook is good. In the debilitated, in drunkards, and in the aged the chances are against recovery. So fatal is it in the latter class (i.e., the elderly) that it has been termed the natural end of the old man."[1]

THE FINAL STAGE: COMFORT CARE AND THE DYING PROCESS

In the latter stage of dementia, independent physical movement slows or even ceases altogether, usually leaving a person bedridden and completely dependent on others. In end-stage dementia, the body begins to shut down, as the brain and nervous system begin to lose their ability to regulate the organs, and the crucial work of the internal organs—breathing, circulation, digestion, elimination, and temperature regulation—slows. Most often, a person in end-stage dementia can no longer swallow and does not respond to offers of food as the body recognizes there is no longer a need to sustain it nutritionally. I have seen people who seem to be otherwise unconscious still tighten their lips to refuse food. Because it is a human tendency to want to encourage someone to eat to sustain life, it can be hard to accept that there comes a time when it is no longer possible for someone to eat or drink. At this time, for most people, care is focused on what is known as "comfort care," or doing anything possible to keep a person comfortable.

Ultimately, the dying process takes over all other functions, entering a stage known as "active dying." Unless there are other medical issues, a person will usually lapse into unconsciousness. Independent movement usually ceases; breathing patterns change; because the ability to swallow is lost, secretions gather in the mouth and throat, leading to a gurgling, liquid sound; usually, the mouth is open to breathe. This ultimate stage can take hours or days, but, generally, a doctor or hospice nurse can make a realistic estimate based on their experience of how long this period will last; no one, however, can predict exactly how long this stage will take.

There are many ways to help keep a dying person comfortable and peaceful. There are special mechanical air mattresses that provide gentle alternations in air pressure, which can help keep a person who is bedridden and immobile from developing bedsores (also known as pressure ulcers); alternatively, caregivers can carefully turn someone who is immobile every few hours for the same purpose. Medications, gentle touch, soft music, mouth care using specially prepared oral swabs to help keep the mouth moist, and offering words of love and support can help soothe and provide some relief. However, when a person in the end stage of dementia no longer takes in food or fluids and the dying process proceeds, their body mechanism slows, finally allowing the natural journey to lead to a usually quiet and peaceful death.

PART II

EXPECTATIONS AND CHALLENGES

CHAPTER THREE

WHAT TO EXPECT

I don't know who you are, but I know I love you.
—grandmother of Gabriela, a young woman who often
visited her grandmother, who was suffering from dementia

While not every case of dementia follows a specific pattern, there are similarities in the way the disease progresses. Generally, as noted earlier, the progression of dementia is described as developing in three stages: mild (or early-stage) dementia, moderate (or middle-stage) dementia, and severe (late- or end-stage) dementia. To make it even more complicated, many dementia scores are rated as mild to moderate or moderate to severe. There is no hard and fast delineation of each stage, but there are signs that can be recognized as belonging to each stage and help indicate what you might expect to come next.

SOMETHING TO THINK ABOUT:
WHEN OTHER ILLNESSES TAKE OVER

While most of this book addresses the progress of dementia and how it inevitably leads to death, some people with dementia die of other things before dementia claims their life. Some people with dementia die from accidents—a person with dementia who wanders into traffic and is hit by a car and dies, dies of the *injury*, although the illness may be a *cause* of the injury—and some die

---

of other diseases, such as a heart attack, diabetes, or cancer. In those cases, they die of another illness before they die of dementia. Whether that is a positive or negative may be difficult to evaluate; however, when those deaths occur, one thing to consider is that the person (and the family) was spared some of the heartbreaking and inevitable decline of dementia.

MILD- OR EARLY-STAGE DEMENTIA

In the early stages of dementia, people often tend to notice by themselves that they are becoming more forgetful. Perhaps your grandmother always sends you a birthday card but later realizes that she forgot this year. Or, when describing a lunch she went to, perhaps she can't remember the name of the person she had lunch with and says something like, "I can't believe it—I see her every week, and I can't think of her name!" She may seem to misplace things like her keys or eyeglasses more frequently and laugh—or berate herself—about it. These small signs begin to add up, and your grandmother may make comments that she's "slipping" or "losing her marbles."

MIDDLE- OR MODERATE-STAGE DEMENTIA

The middle stage of dementia is, in some ways, the most difficult. This stage is a time of increasing disorientation, loss of abilities, and, sometimes, changes in personality. A person in this stage may realize that they are losing their abilities; this can be extremely frightening to them as they begin to recognize their downhill course. They may become quick to anger—whether because of frustration, fear, confusion, or the loss of cells in their brain due to the disease. They may become stubborn, resistant to help, and suspicious of those who try to help them. This is a time when there is a struggle between the desire to maintain their independence and autonomy, and the need to accept help in areas that they can no longer manage.

AL'S STORY: TALKING WITH GRAMMA

Al remembers the early stages of his grandmother's dementia, when she could still engage in meaningful conversations with him. He recalled,

> I remember that one of the first things I noticed, when it was becoming clear that she was often confused about things, was that she was becoming more emotionally needy. When I'd be saying goodbye at the end of a visit, she'd always ask me, "When are you going to visit?" or say, "I'd love it if you did this more often." That was even if I'd been there the day before. It kind of felt insistent, like a sort of anxiousness, that she needed a lot of soothing.
>
> We talked about her condition a lot; she was acknowledging that it was real. She had been a psychologist, so she knew about dementia, and she recognized that her issues with memory were not normal. At that stage, she was able to express her fear, sadness, and even her shame about what was happening to her. That used to make me feel so sad, but it also made me feel lucky that we were able to have those conversations. It was still an equal exchange; there was a lot of openness, and I felt that we still had things to talk about, and I was so glad that we were able to talk about them.

For people in the middle stage of dementia, communication becomes more of an issue. It is often more difficult for them to find the words they are looking for in a conversation. They may have a few stories that they repeat frequently—sometimes during the same conversation or even after a few moments. They may perseverate about things, focusing on a subject, a memory, or something that bothers them, and talk about it again and again, and seem unable to leave it alone. They may have one or two phrases they seem to use often, almost as conversation fillers, for instance, "Well, that's the way it is" or "And so it goes." These are pretty good indications that it's becoming harder for them to focus their thoughts, retrieve words, and participate in and keep track of a conversation.

In the middle stages of dementia, people's interests often become more limited. They may be less interested in activities they used to do; they may be less willing to leave the comfort of their home or join in a social experience. This withdrawal may very well be linked to their knowledge, whether conscious or unconscious, that they are no longer able to "hold their own" in circumstances other than those most familiar and contained. They may feel nervous, scared, or at a loss, because they sense that their ability to take care of themselves is failing. At this stage, my mother would often repeat, over and over again, "I don't know what to do, I don't know what to do."

Because people in mid-stage dementia are becoming disoriented and less sure of themselves, they frequently begin to become paranoid; they may eye people with suspicion; they may accuse someone of stealing something from them, talking about them behind their back, or leaving them out of decisions or events. In fact, sometimes those accusations are true. Family members may be starting to discuss what's going on with Mom or whether they need to take over managing Dad's finances. Because of their increased vulnerability, there very well may be people—family members or household help—who do take advantage of them and misappropriate or steal things from them.

ASSISTIVE DEVICES

As dementia progresses, it is not uncommon for someone to begin to need help when walking, getting up from a chair or off the toilet, or standing or sitting in the bath or shower. Assistive devices are available that can help make these actions easier and safer, and you may see a progression of devices in the house as disability increases. From using a cane to using a walker and from pushing a personal shopping cart (often referred to as a "Granny cart") to using a rollator (a more elaborate walker that may include a basket and can convert to a seat), people begin to need these devices to navigate day-to-day life. They may "graduate" from being able to walk with a walker to needing to be pushed in a wheelchair. There are implements that can be used to raise toilet seats, making it easier for someone to sit and stand. Grab bars can be installed in bathtubs or showers and along bathroom walls, providing secure handholds and hopefully preventing falls. Bedrails can offer support so patients can pull themselves up in bed, and poles can help them stand from a sitting position. Bedside commodes allow someone to eliminate without having to walk or be wheeled to a bathroom toilet. Handles can assist someone in rising from a chair, and mechanical or electrically operated "lift recliners" can raise someone from a sitting to a standing position when they can no longer do it themselves. These devices can help extend the time that a person can remain mobile and safe, as the disease saps their muscle strength, balance, and stability. While not considered "assistive devices," many people will need to wear "adult diapers" when they are no longer able to depend on their bladder or bowel control.

Unfortunately, many of these devices are expensive. Some of them may be covered by insurance when prescribed by a doctor or other medical professional. Many may be too costly for an individual or family to afford. There are charitable organizations that accept donations of used equipment and provide them at no cost to people who need them. You can help search for available equipment by checking with churches, synagogues, or senior centers and looking online for local organizations that may be able to link you to such resources.

SEVERE-, LATE-, OR END-STAGE DEMENTIA

Late-stage dementia is when, in some senses, things become both more difficult and easier. They become more difficult because the issues of care become more complex, the needs of the individual are harder to manage, and the downward decline is heartrending and sad to observe. In some ways, however, things become easier because the individual with dementia generally becomes more passive, more apathetic, and less able to be argumentative or resistant. They also lose some sense of understanding or consciousness of their situation, although—sometimes, and heartbreakingly—there often does seem to be awareness, even sadness, behind the most blank of expressions. But this is also a time when it can be easier for you to provide tender, loving attention in the most basic ways—holding a hand, stroking an arm, talking or singing softly, and just *being there* for them.

BATHING AND CLEANLINESS

Personal hygiene becomes a problem as a person with dementia begins to be unable to take care of their own needs. By this stage, people are occasionally, and in come cases totally, incontinent (unable to control their urinary or bowel functions). They probably require complete assistance with toileting or need to have adult diapers changed. Bathing becomes more difficult to manage; sometimes the issues stem from such physical challenges as difficulty stepping into a bathtub or being unable to raise their arms over their head to wash their hair; more often the challenge is not physical, but due to mental decline and the emotional stressors that go along with it.

SOMETHING TO THINK ABOUT: WHY BATHING CAN BE A BATTLEGROUND

Bathing is often a moment of disturbance and agitation for someone who has dementia. Consider that—for almost all of us—bathing, showering, and brushing your teeth are intensely private times. We are generally used to privacy when changing our clothes or using the restroom, and we have our habits and ways of doing things. For someone who needs assistance and is used to a certain modesty about their bodies and bodily functions, having someone—whether it be a family member, nurse, or home-care aide—come into the bathroom with them, remove their clothes, and begin to try to get them to step into the bath or shower, can be a frightening, invasive, overwhelming experience. So they may respond in the only way they can—by arguing, fighting back, pushing, crying, or refusing to be moved.

Contributing to this emotional experience, also consider that bathrooms are generally a place of hard, shiny, bright surfaces and light; we design bathrooms with mirrors, glossy tiles, and bright lighting to see ourselves reflected clearly in the mirrors. While we can enjoy these polished finishes when we are healthy, they can contribute to sensory shock on the part of someone with dementia.

Other issues that contribute to the tension of bath time are fears of drowning or scalding, due to changes in how someone with dementia senses temperature and touch. Even if someone is not able to consciously recognize these fears, they can rise to the surface when someone who is already confused becomes agitated.

SOMETHING TO THINK ABOUT: THE DELICATE BALANCE OF HELPING WITH PERSONAL HYGIENE

While you may not be the person who helps your grandparent bathe, there are things you can think about and even suggest to help make the process more comfortable and less distressing. Consider, first of all, the issue of modesty and the ramifications of intergenerational discomfort with assistance with personal hygiene. At some point, you may be the one who helps your grandmother with personal care, whether assisting her to the toilet or helping her to wash or bathe. Your grandmother may be distressed by the need to have you attend her at such a private moment, and you may be distressed for the same reason. But this can also be a profoundly significant moment for you both.

Author Jean Kwok wrote about it sensitively in her recent novel *Searching for Sylvie Lee*, when a young woman must help her grandmother with personal care:

I escorted her to the toilet and bath, exposing pale skin untouched by the sun, arms and legs grown so spindly and frail, an intimacy she had never shared with me before. Grandma's chin had trembled the first time, but I said, "When you love someone, there is no shame. When I see you, I only know that you are my grandma and you are beautiful. You did this for me when I was young. Now it is my turn. You always said the old become children once again."

If it has become clear that bathing is something your grandmother resists, it may be better not to announce it, for instance, by saying, "I'm going to help you take a shower now." It is best to prepare the bathing materials—towels, soap, shampoo, bathmat, tub mat, or shower chair—before bringing your grandmother into the bathroom. Pick a time for bathing when she is calm, perhaps with quiet music on in the background, and see if she can be gently led or brought into the bathroom as part of a "walk," a "little stroll," or even a gentle dance movement. Crooning speech, a little song, soothing stroking, a gentle back rub, or patting motions might help ease the transition to bathing.

Offer soap or shampoo to smell as a sensory pleasure, suggesting how delicious they smell or what they smell like, for example, "Doesn't this smell like a green apple?" or "I love how this smells like vanilla." Offer a washcloth to hold, or encourage them to help clean themselves to include your loved one in the activity. As long as every means is used to ensure safety in the bathroom, try to encourage their participation as much as possible.

Sometimes agitation and fear can be lessened through talking softly, moving and touching gently and soothingly, and using dimmer lights so that harsh lighting doesn't cause glare. Use soft washcloths and warm water, and always try to make the experience soothing rather than shocking. Make sure that there are no slippery surfaces on the bathroom floor or in the shower or tub and that there are solid grab bars in place, and make every effort to create a serene and safe space.

AGITATION

Many people who have dementia have episodes of agitation. This can be a physical manifestation of their disease, but also an expression of their heightened worries and frustrations. They may have periods of being unable to sit still, walk or pace endlessly, or start to flail their arms or try to kick, and their ability to listen to reason or calm themselves can disappear. The agitation that often accompanies dementia can be self-perpetuating. People with dementia lose the ability to regulate their emotions and behavior, so that while healthy people might be able to catch themselves when they are getting upset and readjust their emotions and thinking to pull themselves together, very often that is beyond the abilities of someone with dementia.

SOMETHING TO THINK ABOUT: PHYSICAL CAUSES OF AGITATION

When a person with dementia starts to become fidgety or agitated, consider whether there may be a physical discomfort that they cannot verbally articulate and can only express through agitation. Do they need to use the toilet and perhaps have already soiled themselves? Are they too hot or too cold? Are they sitting comfortably, or is something causing them discomfort, for example, an arm squeezed against an armrest, or is a cushion or piece of clothing bunched uncomfortably beneath them? Are they hungry or tired of sitting upright and want to lay down? If a physical cause can be identified and alleviated, that can reduce the distress. If you or others in the family or caregiver circle can learn to read the signs, it can reduce the likelihood of persistent distress.

SPEECH AND COMMUNICATION DIFFICULTIES

Dysphasia is the loss of or deficiency in the power to use or understand language as a result of injury to or disease of the brain.[2] As
dementia progresses, the ability to speak becomes compromised,
known as dysphasia. Your grandfather may no longer be able to put
words together in a sentence; he may struggle more to find a word. He
may use a word that does not seem to make sense or repeat a word over
and over again. He may echo a word that you said and repeat it again
and again or repeat the last word of every sentence you say. He may be

WHEN COMMUNICATION IS
EXPRESSED THROUGH TOUCH

"When I volunteered at a day program for people with dementia, I
spent a lot of my time with one woman," Hattie, a young volunteer,
recalled. "She was nonverbal, but she loved to touch me. She would
sit there next to me, and she would stroke my hand, she would hold
my hand, she would stroke my hair, touch my face, kiss my hand.
She was expressing affection and how much she appreciated my
being with her."

Khadija, another young volunteer at a nursing home, pointed
out that, "Holding hands helps. Sometimes a resident I'm with
doesn't want to talk or can't talk, and we'll sit outside and be quiet.
But then they might put their hand on the arm of their chair, and
I'll reach over to hold it, and we'll just sit there together like that."

Navya, who works with Khadija, echoed the same senitment.
"It's like you're present in the moment, and you give them that
touch, and it's like, Okay, I'm here with you. Sometimes they love
it when you go up to them and give them a high five," she reflected.
"It's like a reminder that they're not alone. Some of them, coming
to live here in the nursing home, they definitely feel lonely. So
having someone next to them, just the fact of touching them, and
giving them some attention, it's huge."

frustrated and become agitated by this inability to communicate, or he may not seem bothered or aware of it at all.

For some people with advancing dementia, this stage is marked by such nonverbal vocalizations as repeating a sound or syllable—"ba, ba, ba, ba, ba," for instance. In some people, it manifests as grunting or repeating the name of a loved one over and over again—sometimes louder and louder until it's almost yelling. It can be particularly heart-rending when someone with severe dementia is distressed or agitated and cries or screams incoherently and seems inconsolable. This may be partly because they *can't* express whatever it is that bothers them, but sometimes it is a symptom of the disease and seems to have no apparent cause at all.

RAMIE'S SOLUTION: FINDING A COMMON LANGUAGE

Ramie, a young man who volunteers at a nursing home, recalled an experience that highlighted the value of trying to meet a person on their level. Said Ramie,

> There was this one lady; she didn't talk to anybody. All she did was grunt at people. One day, I was taking her outside to sit in the garden, and I tried to start a conversation with her. But whenever I would say something, she wouldn't say anything back, all she'd do is kind of grunt, make a kind of a "ruh, ruh" sound. So, I just found myself making the same sound back at her—not to make fun of her, but to show her that I understood what she was saying. She looked starstruck! So, then we just had a conversation going in grunting. She seemed happy and seemed to respond to it. But then, when I asked her if she wanted to go upstairs, I was totally amazed when she said, "Yeah"—perfectly fine!

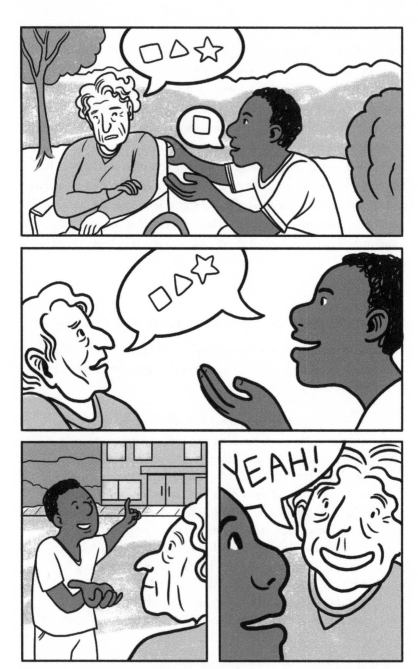

When volunteering at the nursing home, Ramie would converse with one of the dementia patients by repeating the sounds she made. *Illustration by Kate Haberer*

LOSS OF RECOGNITION: WHEN GRANDMA NO LONGER RECOGNIZES YOU

Loss of recognition is a particularly hard but almost inevitable stage in the course of dementia. You may hardly notice when it begins; perhaps your grandmother no longer greets you by name, although she may still seem happy to see you. She may call you by your mother's name; your sister's name; or that of her own, long-dead sister. While this may be distressing to you, it is often the case that, while she may not know who you are, your grandmother does retain the sense that you and she are close, and that you are important to her. It is at this stage that some of the most poignant—and meaningful—moments are felt. As one young woman, Gabriela, told me, with tears in her eyes, every single time she went to visit her grandmother, Nana, in the last few years of her life, her grandmother would hug her and say, "I don't know who you are, but I know I love you."

CHAPTER FOUR

WHAT YOU CAN DO TO HELP SOMEONE WITH DEMENTIA

It's important to just go with the flow.
—Khadija, young volunteer

*There is a moral task of caregiving, and that involves just being there,
being with that person and being committed. When there is nothing that
can be done, we have to be able to say, "Look, I'm with you in this experience. Right through to the end of it."*

In many ways, just being there is the most profound, most generous,
and most meaningful thing you can do for someone who has
dementia. Whether it is sitting in silence, reading aloud, singing
together, or looking at photographs together, your physical presence—
your "being there"—is the greatest gift you can offer.

Helping someone continue to feel that they have a meaningful
place in life, in *your* life, can be a wonderful thing to share. Seeing
someone who feels they have no purpose left in life can be hard. As Amy
Tan wrote in her novel *The Bonesetter's Daughter*, "It broke her heart to
see her mother trying so hard, being so conscientious, so determined
to be valuable. . . . LuLing simply wanted to be essential, as a mother
should be."[1]

There are many things you can do that have not only meaningful but useful and comforting benefits for someone with dementia. There are some things to consider that may have adverse effects on someone with dementia, and it is helpful to know what those are so that you can help keep life as calm and enjoyable as possible during what can be a tumultuous time.

SLOW THINGS DOWN

Young people generally speak and move more quickly than older people. Recognize that your beloved grandfather is not only moving slower than he used to, but also that his ability to think clearly, hear words, and make sense of them is also slowing. It can be helpful to slow down—both in movement and speech—to be less disconcerting to him. Meet him "in his space" and try to pace yourself to his level of comfort. Pay attention to how he seems to be processing what you say or whether he seems befuddled by your activity.

BE A MORE EFFECTIVE COMMUNICATOR: LOW AND SLOW

In an earlier section, I discuss the issue of hearing loss in older people. While some people may have hearing aids that enable them to hear, following a conversation still can be difficult, especially for someone with some dementia.

One important thing to remember is that yelling does not help. Moreover, raising your voice can be perceived as being rude or intentionally offensive. There are several tricks to using your speaking voice to help you be better heard and understood:

- Pitch your voice a little lower. For many people with hearing loss, higher voices are more difficult to hear. If you lower the pitch of your voice, you may find you are more easily heard and understood. (Pitch is not about loudness; it is about whether you speak with a *high* voice or a *low* voice; try saying a few words as you normally would, and then try to say them with a lower, deeper voice.)

- While you certainly shouldn't yell, it may help to speak in a slightly louder, clearer voice than you might in normal conversation. Watch for physical signs that you might be speaking too loudly: If the person pulls back or squeezes their eyes shut for a moment as though to shut out a sound, that's probably a sign that you are speaking more loudly than you should.

- Speak more slowly. Young people tend to speak fast—and you may not even realize you are doing it. Make a conscious effort to talk a little more slowly than you usually would, and keep your sentences simple and straightforward.

- When speaking, make sure your listener can watch your face. People with hearing loss, whether or not they also have dementia, can often piece together what you are saying, even if they miss a few words, if they are watching your face.

- A simpler, less expensive alternative to hearing aids are *personal hearing amplifiers*, which are available in pharmacies or where small electronics are sold. Personal hearing amplifiers are usually headphones connected to a small amplifier that can be worn on a cord around the person's neck. While they are not as effective as hearing aids, they can offer some improvement in hearing, which can make an important difference to someone with dementia.

DON'T ARGUE WITH, CORRECT, EMBARRASS, DEMEAN, OR INFANTILIZE THE PERSON WITH DEMENTIA

One of the hardest things to handle when you love someone with dementia is to hear them say something wrong, hear them repeat something over and over again, or see them do something inappropriate. It can be hard not to get short-tempered or annoyed when a person with dementia insists on something that you know to be incorrect or nonsensical. They can be repetitive; they can ask the same question over and over; they can say something that does not make sense or is outright incorrect. Very often a person with dementia will refuse to believe something you tell them. Sometimes their behavior or something they say can seem childish, embarrassing, or even insulting or hurtful.

It can be very hard, at times, not to snap back, and it can be difficult not to take a hurtful comment personally. Try to keep in mind that *it is the disease* that is causing those comments or that behavior, and your grandfather *cannot control* or modulate what he is saying or doing. Trying to insist on your version might only cause him to become argumentative, upset, or even belligerent. Unless it is a matter of ensuring his imminent safety, it is usually better not to try to convince him or argue with him about reality. Accept that *his* view of reality may be different from *actual* reality, and he needs to maintain his belief. It is generally better to back off a bit and see whether you can change the subject, agree with him, or just let things go. Keeping the atmosphere calm and balanced is usually the best path to follow.

JOSEF'S STORY: GOING ALONG AND GETTING ALONG

At the nursing home where I volunteer, I was assigned to take this one woman outside to the garden in her wheelchair. When I told her I was there to take her out, she firmly told me no, that she didn't want to go. So I just walked away for a minute. When I came back and introduced myself again and told her we were going to go out. She'd forgotten that she'd said no before, and she said okay. While I was wheeling her out, she told me that she used to live in Queens, New York, and we had a conversation about where she used to live. But then she started saying, "I want to go home." I didn't want to make her sad, so I said, "Okay, we're going to go back to Queens," and we talked a little more about Queens. A little later, when I began to wheel her back indoors, she asked, "We're going to Queens?" and I said, "Yeah, we're going to go to Queens," and she seemed happy. It was time to take her upstairs for lunch, and I wasn't sure how she'd react, but when I took her into the dining room, she looked around and said, "I love it here!" It was like her mood changed, just like that. Now, every time I see her, I greet her with, "We're going to go to Queens," and she says, "Yes, we're going to Queens!" with a big smile on her face. I felt it made her happy to think she was going to Queens, even if she only remembered for a minute. It made her feel good, and she was in a good place. It just sometimes takes improvisation.

A PROFESSIONAL'S ADVICE: UNDERSTAND THE EMOTIONS BEHIND THE WORDS

I recently spoke with Grace, a social worker who works with people with dementia and their families. When I asked Grace why she chose that field, she explained that her interest grew from her close relationship with and love for her grandmother, who died from dementia while Grace was in high school. Grace recalled one particular incident that unnerved her when she was young. One day, when she walked in to visit her grandmother, her grandmother began to cry out to her, over and over again, "You have to take me! You have to take me! I have to go to the wedding!" It so distressed Grace that she went into the other room and burst out crying.

I asked Grace how, knowing what she knows now through her education and experience, she might have handled the situation differently. She said,

Of course, I wouldn't have known this as a teenager, but I think what I would do now is try to understand what was going on with my grandmother, why was she starting to get anxious. It's all about validation, asking questions, validating the emotions behind the

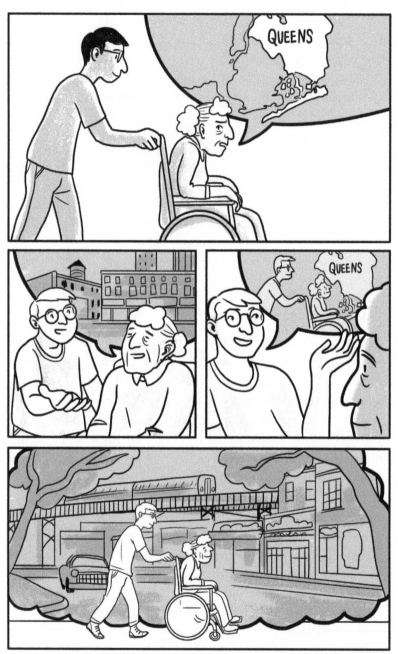

Josef would wheel the woman out to the garden and talk about going to Queens, where she grew up, which made her happy and calm. *Illustration by Kate Haberer*

words. Even if the words don't make sense, you need to recognize that those emotions are real. She was clearly feeling some urgency, a sense that something needed to happen. Even if you can't understand the words or if they don't make sense—if they're what we call "word salad"—then you can try to hear the emotions behind them and respond to those, so you're meeting them at that moment. That's what people need when they're in a high emotional state; they want someone to listen and to be there with them. So now, perhaps, I might ask her about the details, try to ask her about the wedding, maybe get her reminiscing about her wedding. I'd gently try to redirect the conversation in a related way. I also know now that it's *not* always possible to redirect someone, so I would try to soothe or even go along with her thoughts and words if I could.

ENCOURAGE AND SUPPORT INDEPENDENCE

A person with cognitive decline will inevitably experience the loss of independence and control. As they become less able to handle day-to-day functions, less able to take care of their own needs, and necessarily more reliant on others—whether family or paid caregivers—most people find it difficult, if not intolerable, to give up that autonomy and control. They can and often will fight against accepting help, even when it is clearly needed. It is for this reason that it becomes increasingly important to allow them to do for themselves whatever they can do. Sometimes a caregiver takes over an activity—feeding, dressing, or even doing a puzzle—because it is easier or quicker to do it than to enable the person with dementia to participate or do it for themselves. One thing you can do is try to support and encourage your loved one to do as much as they can for themselves, and even make it easier for them to do so if possible. Keep in mind, though, that while support and encouragement can be good, letting someone struggle to do something they are unable to do can be frustrating and lead to an agitated or aggressive response.

DEAL THOUGHTFULLY WITH AGITATION AND DISTRESS

When someone becomes upset, the first step should be to attempt to take the emotions down a notch if you can. Back off—both physically and verbally. Take a step back and try to speak slowly, softly, and reassuringly, without being condescending—very often someone with dementia is exquisitely sensitive to recognizing condescension. Sometimes, however, these techniques don't work. Try to change the subject or divert their attention, even with something as simple as asking if they'd like a drink of water or want to take a walk. Step away to take the pressure off; agree with them. If it's safe to do so, step out of the room and return, as though nothing happened, and start again—with a change of subject. The upside of dementia is that things are quickly forgotten, and a mood can change in an instant.

A CREATIVE WAY TO DEFLECT A TENSE SITUATION

Carmen was the longtime aide to Mrs. M, the 101-year-old matriarch of a loving family. Carmen had a gentle, warm, and sensitive relationship with Mrs. M, whom she always kept beautifully groomed and dressed, although Mrs. M was no longer able to speak or recognize those she loved.

One morning, when Carmen arrived for her daytime shift and went to greet Mrs. M, Mrs. M became agitated and started crying out, "Get away! Who are you? Get out of my house!" At first, Carmen gently tried to remind her who she was, but she quickly realized that Mrs. M was past the point of being calmed by talking to her. So, Carmen backed away, said goodbye to Mrs. M, and left the room for a few minutes. She took off her coat and put on an apron so she would look different. She then walked back into the room where Mrs. M was sitting and—as though nothing had happened and the day was starting all over again—greeted Mrs. M cheerfully, bustling around to make breakfast. Mrs. M's face brightened, and she smiled, her agitation having disappeared.

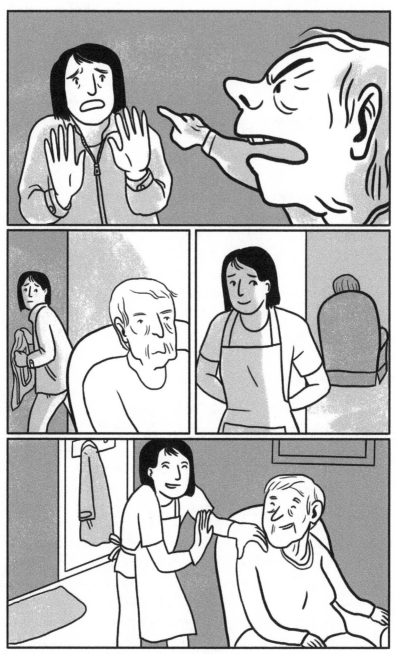

Mrs. M was agitated when Carmen came in one morning, so Carmen said goodbye, put on an apron, and tried again. This time, Mrs. M was happy to see her and greeted her cheerfully. *Illustration by Kate Haberer*

USE HELPFUL REMINDERS

When a person's memory is beginning to fade but they are still able to maintain some independence in their daily life, some simple things can be done to help jog their memory.

POST NOTES

A chalkboard, whiteboard, bulletin board, or even sticky notes placed in a clearly visible spot, for instance, the inner side of the front door or on the refrigerator, can be updated regularly with such things as appointments or even reminders like, "Check that you've turned off the stove" or "Remember to take your keys." Just make sure that if you help prepare such reminders that your grandparent does not feel insulted by them. One way to do that might be to include them in writing and posting the notes.

KEEP CALENDAR UP-TO-DATE

A large calendar with space to write down important dates can be something you consult and update together. Checking the calendar with your grandmother is also a way to help orient her to the date and day of the week, which often get confused when dementia sets in.

WRITE EXPLANATORY NOTES

Grace, a social worker who works with people with dementia in a nursing home, told me about a woman who began to ask the staff over and over again, "Where's my daughter?" No matter how many times they would answer her, she would ask again. On an index card, Grace wrote, "Your daughter is fine. Your daughter is at work. Your daughter will come to visit around 5 o'clock," and she helped the woman put the card in her purse. Whenever she would ask about her daughter, the staff would remind her to look at her card. Although this measure didn't put a stop to her questioning, it reduced the number of times per hour that she repeated her question and kept her calmer. "It gave her some control over the information," Grace explained.

BRING YOUR YOUTH, JOY, AND SENSE OF FUN TO THE MOMENT

Remember that your energy and youthful zest can be a wonderful tonic to someone with dementia. I recognize that it can be hard and sometimes exhausting to spend time with a person whose mind and body are in decline, but think about what you can bring to them and what a difference you can make in their day. Before you visit with your grandparent, think about summoning that energy and natural enthusiasm, and bring it in with you. You'll find that you can more easily start things off on a lively note.

EDELYSA'S METHOD

Edelysa worked as a teen volunteer in high school and college, and is now supervising teen volunteers who work in the memory care unit of a nursing home. Many of the residents there are in the late stages of dementia; most are wheelchair-bound, many are barely verbal or entirely nonverbal, and many appear passive or nonresponsive. Said Edelysa,

> I remember the first day I started. An older volunteer took me around, and he showed me the various floors where I'd be working. Then, when we got into the elevator, one man who was wandering the halls tried to get onto the elevator with us and got pretty disruptive when they tried to prevent him from doing that. It was kind of scary, and I'm like, "Whoa, this is what I signed up for?" But then, once I started and got some experience, the dementia floor became my favorite floor to work on. The people there get

so excited to see me, they seem to perk up, and it becomes fun for me; it changed my whole perspective.

Now, when I head up to that floor, there's always music playing, and I walk in bopping, snapping my fingers, and I kind of dance my way in with a big smile on my face. They laugh and try to dance along with me, even the people who are in wheelchairs, and I always get a smile or some great reaction. I feel so good to be able to bring that positive energy to them.

USE MUSIC

Music can function in many ways as a tool for helping someone with dementia. Music can be a soothing background and an entertaining activity, and it can help spark memories and conversation. Music can be a diversion when someone with dementia begins to get distressed, agitated, or argumentative. It can help calm things down, or it can help liven things up. Whether you have any musical abilities yourself hardly matters. There are numerous ways to incorporate music into a visit, and for someone with dementia, your being able to carry a tune or play an instrument without mistakes may make less difference than it does to someone whose cognitive abilities are unimpaired.

JANE'S STORY: HOW MUSIC MADE A DIFFERENCE

Jane, a highly accomplished young pianist, volunteered in high school for an organization that sends professional and student musicians into the homes of homebound people to provide concert-level performances. Jane recalled one early visit to a frail, elderly gentleman who had had a long and distinguished career in the music industry, and suffered from Lewy body dementia, a type of progressive cognitive decline that can also severely impair physical movement. Wheelchair bound, the gentleman could barely move or speak. "The first visit was the most memorable for me," Jane recounted.

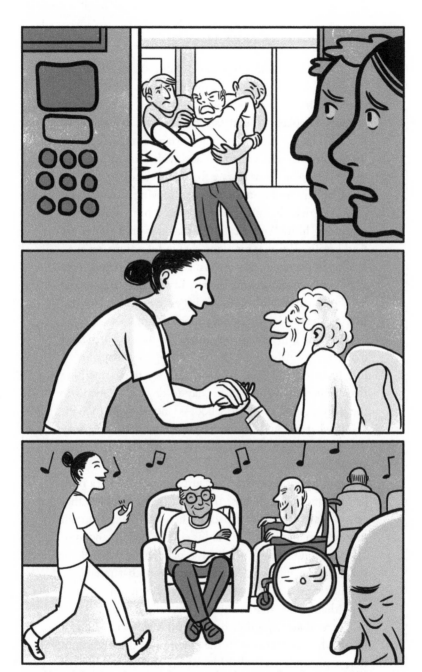

Even though her first day was a bit scary, the dementia floor became Edelysa's favorite place to volunteer. *Illustration by Kate Haberer*

I was there with my trio—a violinist, a cellist, and me—and we played the first movement of a piece. I didn't think we had played very well, but when we'd finished playing, I looked up and saw that he was struggling to move his hands—he was trying to clap for us, which was incredible. His wife was there, and with tears in her eyes, she told us that it was so rare for him to make any movement at all. It was tremendously moving because you could see that the music had animated him, and he was expressing himself physically. So that was pretty amazing. And I realized, at that moment, that it did not matter at all how I was playing, because the meaningfulness came from us being there and sharing the music with him. Because he had been surrounded by music his entire career, this visit, hearing the music, profoundly affected him.

Visiting him and playing music for him made me feel like I was contributing to his well-being, to his quality of life. It was an amazing experience to see that something that seemed so intrinsic in my day-to-day life—practicing the piano, going to music school—I never really thought about what it could do for other people. Seeing the way that it manifested in his reaction—it was very profound, an unforgettable experience.

During another visit, I had just finished playing a Bach prelude and fugue. I chose that piece because I knew that one of his specialties was Bach. When I finished, I turned toward him and his wife, and his aide looked up and said, "He was conducting!" While I was playing, he was making small movements with his hand in a way that resembled conducting. That was another incredible moment, realizing that he was able to connect with the Bach.

It reminded me that he was still a person, a human being who connected with the emotion of the music and that it probably reminded him of his passion throughout his life. Despite his condition, he was still able to demonstrate that he felt tied to the music. That was illuminating for me. Before volunteering for the program, I had never encountered anyone with dementia, and it was just very profound to see evidence of a continued sense of living, even though their condition inhibits them in so many ways.

One of the most amazing things is how someone whose cognitive abilities have already diminished so much that they may not even be able to speak, or at least not to speak in any organized way, can suddenly carry a tune and even sing the words to songs they knew long ago. Many times, the areas of the brain that control musical memory and the ability to recall the lyrics to a song remain functional long after the areas that control spoken words have lost the ability to function.

Music therapy is a special therapeutic technique that, for someone with dementia, can involve using music in many forms to help retrieve memories, encourage speech, soothe, enliven, and simply provide pleasure. Music therapists are trained in how to use music—instrumental, recorded, and vocal—interactively to engage and support the cognitive, emotional, and physical areas that lose elasticity and function in those with dementia.

Even without training as a music therapist, there are ways in which any of us can use music to help someone with dementia. One of the simplest ways is to play recorded music, whether on the radio, a CD player, your computer, or even your cell phone.

SOMETHING TO THINK ABOUT: HOW SOUNDS CAN BE DISTRESSING

Many people with dementia process sound more slowly and with more difficulty than when they were healthy. Sounds, even music, can be perceived as jangly—annoying, agitating, distressing.

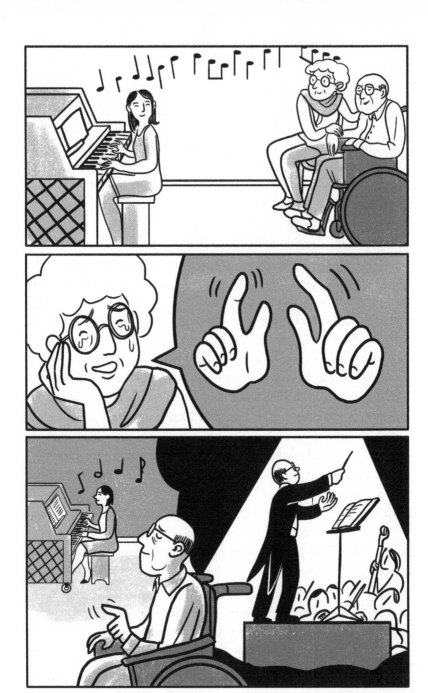

Jane played piano for a retired conductor; due to dementia, he could hardly move. But when Jane played Bach, his hands would move like he was conducting because he still connected so deeply with the music. *Illustration by Kate Haberer*

Sometimes this can be prevented by playing music softly or not using music as a background to conversation. It can also be harder for someone with cognitive decline to understand what someone is saying while music is playing; I generally try to avoid conversation if there is background music unless the music is very soft.

Try to find music that would be enjoyable for the person with dementia. Do you know if they preferred classical music or popular? Instrumental or vocal? Do you know any particular favorites they always liked? Keep in mind that the music is not for *you*; you don't have to like what you play for them. Not an opera fan but Gramma always was? Play her favorite. You might learn something about opera and start to appreciate it yourself. If she's able to speak, ask her about opera and why she loves it or what it means to her; it can be a joy for both of you.

HELP MAKE VISITS MORE COMFORTABLE

For someone in the later stages of dementia, sounds and noises can sometimes cause frightening cognitive dissonance. Having more than one person talking at a time or joining in a conversation can be extremely agitating. When possible, I always tried to arrange for only one person to visit my mother at a time. I found that if two or three (or even more) people tried to have a conversation with her, she would either seem to "shut down," blanking out as though she was trying to escape from the chatter, or begin to get agitated. It's not always easy to arrange this; visitors sometimes arrive together, parents want to bring their children, or out-of-town relatives want to visit Grampa at the same time. One way to lessen the confusion for Grandpa might be to have only one person sit with him at a time, with the others waiting their turn in another room. If there must be multiple people in the room at the same time, try not to have overlapping conversations or more than one person speaking at once. But when trying to limit overlapping conversation, do so tactfully; you don't want to offend anyone, you're just trying to make a good thing better.

PARTICIPATE OR JOIN IN ACTIVITIES

If your grandmother attends a day program at a senior center, see if you can bring her or visit her there; she may get enjoyment from showing you off to her friends or showing you "her place" or "her friends." If she gets or goes to physical therapy sessions, for example, see if you can be there occasionally; it will give you insight into what is being done for her, and you may also pick up some pointers on things you can do to help. Being present for such opportunities gives your grandmother the chance to introduce you and interact with others about you. These can be meaningful social connections that help include her in daily life.

HELP MAKE PHONE CONVERSATIONS EASIER

Talking on the phone can be an important way to maintain contact and interaction with someone with dementia, and offer them bright spots in their day. However, as dementia progresses, phone conversations can become difficult. Your grandmother may not be able to visualize or understand who is on the other end of the phone line; it is helpful to identify who is speaking. If you're the one who's calling your grandmother, don't assume she'll recognize your voice. Preface the conversation with, "Hi, Grandma, it's me, your grandson, John." If you happen to be with her when she gets a call, offer to answer the phone for her and explain to her who's calling before she begins speaking with them. If she is not able to hear clearly, make sure her hearing aids are in place if she needs them and the phone sound level is as high as it can be. There are also specially designed phones (both landline and mobile) with larger buttons and numerals, simpler functions, and more audible sound, specially made for people with hearing loss or cognitive deficits;

if possible and appropriate, see if your grandmother might be able to get or use one.

MAKE AND POST A SIMPLE PHONE LIST

Phone calls are a wonderful connection for someone with dementia, but placing a call can become confusing for someone suffering from this disease. Your grandfather may have forgotten phone numbers he has always known by heart, misplaced or thrown out his phone book, or forgotten how to look up the names of people he'd like to call. One thing you can do to help is create a simple, large-type list of the names, numbers, and brief identification (for example, "Bob, oldest son" or "Tom, best friend") for the five to ten people he'd most likely call, and post it next to the telephone. This handy list will be helpful for not only your grandfather, but also for anyone else, such as a home aide, who might place a call or answer the phone for him.

TRY TO MINIMIZE CONVERSATIONAL CONFUSION

For someone who is beginning to have difficulty organizing their thoughts or making decisions, being confronted by an open-ended question ("What would you like to do today?" or "What would you like to eat?") can overwhelm them and make them more confused, or even make them agitated. It is usually more effective, and less distressing, to give a simple, two-part choice ("Would you like soup or a peanut butter sandwich?" or "Would you like to go for a walk or play cards?"). Similarly, you can help encourage a conversation with a targeted question rather than something general: For instance, rather than asking, "What do you remember from when you were a child?" ask something that might help jog their memory, like, "Did you play baseball with your friends when you were a little boy?"

USE FRIENDLY REMINDERS TO AVOID CONFUSION

When someone is beginning to forget familiar faces, it is not only helpful, but also *kind* to give them a gentle, friendly reminder. Long before my mother became confused about who I was, I began a habit of identifying myself humorously every time I walked in. "Hi, Mom, it's me, Jean, your one-and-only daughter," I'd call out, or, "Good morning, Mom, it's me, Jean, your favorite and smartest daughter." I hoped it would both remind her of my name and who I was, and start my visit on a light-hearted note (she knew I was her *only* daughter!), forestalling any chance that she might be distressed not to know who I was.

If there is anyone else with you, whether an aide, a family member, or a friend, be aware that your grandmother's ability to recognize them may falter even during a short visit. To be helpful, use their name or describe who they are or why they are there ("She's Annie, your helper, and she's making lunch for you now" or "Isn't it nice that my friend, Sandy, came to visit you today?").

TAKE YOUR CUES FROM THE PERSON WITH DEMENTIA

Like anyone else, someone with cognitive decline has changing moods. It may be beneficial to distract someone who is upset and distressed or try to reduce their agitation; such moods can be disruptive or destructive. Other moods can be valid expressions of feeling, and you should consider taking your cues from your grandparents and try to accept and respect their moods, and go along as they change. Be sensitive of their feelings, whether or not they can verbally express them. As Khadija, a young volunteer, says, "It's important to just go with the flow."

HATTIE'S STORY: PERSISTENCE PAYS OFF

Hattie is a young woman whose work as a volunteer with people in various stages of cognitive decline has fueled her interest in pursuing the study of dementia in the future. Her earliest experience with people with dementia was when she became a volunteer with a program called Sweet Readers, which pairs middle-school students with older people with dementia to explore and create art, music, poetry, and dance as they get to know one another. Said Hattie,

> When I started working with people with dementia, I began to see how isolating the disease is. When people begin to lose the ability to communicate, they get very frustrated; they may be trying hard to be understood, and when they're not, they sometimes get angry and even aggressive. It's not that they're a bad person; it's that the disease is making them frustrated.
>
> I would visit this one person every week; she always seemed to be very angry and, in the beginning, didn't even seem like she wanted my company and didn't want to participate in the activities. She could be verbally aggressive and sometimes seemed to be on the verge of physical aggression; the other volunteers didn't want to work with her. As I came to know her more over the weeks, I realized that she was mostly just sad and frustrated. She was very particular about whom she would agree to partner with, but I decided I wanted to partner with her and was pretty persistent about it. You had to be very careful about what you would say to her; she was an artist, and if we were working on an art project together, she wouldn't hesitate to say my work was awful. Then she would want to show me her work from the past, which she carried in her pocketbook—she wouldn't touch a brush or a pencil to draw anymore, but she liked to show me her work and tell me about it. She was fierce, but I enjoyed being with her; I found it more of a challenge but, at the same time, much more rewarding when I'd get a good reaction from her.

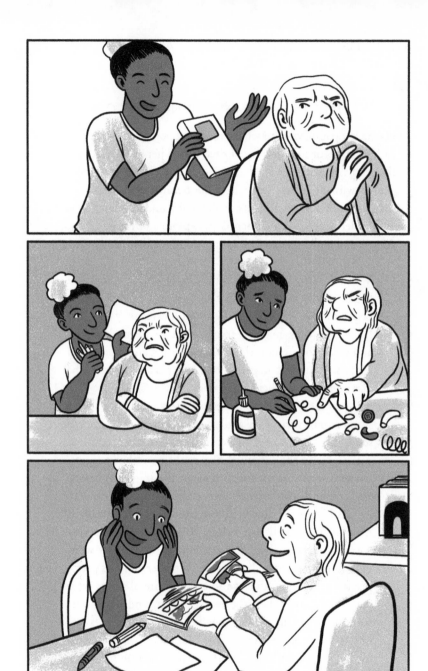

One of the women with whom Hattie volunteered was always angry and aggressive. But as Hattie continued to work with her, the woman warmed up and proudly showed her the artwork she had made in the past. *Illustration by Kate Haberer*

BE IN THE MOMENT

Sometimes the best moment to be in is the present one, and sometimes it is the past; sometimes, it is best to be lively and upbeat, and sometimes it is better to be quiet, empathetic, and calm. Sometimes it is valuable to acknowledge the present moment, but sometimes it can be helpful to let yourself slip into the past with your loved one, to let them live in the memory as though it is the present. If your grandmother mistakes you for her child, or her sister or brother, or thinks you are her mother, you don't need to correct her, and you can even go along with her, share in her reality without playacting, and use it to draw out memories and conversation. If she asks, for example, "Mama, why aren't you cooking dinner yet?" rather than answering, "But Gramma, I'm not your mother, I'm your granddaughter, and it's only 10 o'clock in the morning!" it can be less distressing to her to respond with something like, "What do you think you might like for dinner?" and see if you can engage her in a related conversation.

JOSEF'S WORDS OF WISDOM

Josef, a young volunteer in the memory care unit of a nursing home, had this to say about his experience:

There's a magic that happens between me and an older person with dementia. They see a spark in your eye, a smile on your face, and that's something healing, something that you're bringing to them.

When you walk into the room with people with dementia and you make that connection, it doesn't have to be verbal communication. You bring that smile, that positive energy, that willingness to be in the moment with them, to get at who they are; at this moment, it may not be who they were sixty or seventy years ago, but it's what they need now.

ASK YOUR GRANDPARENT
TO TEACH YOU SOMETHING

As mentioned earlier, oftentimes, in later years, people feel that they no longer have a meaningful role in life. One thing you can do to help them feel that they indeed still have important things to offer is to ask your grandparents to teach you something. If your grandmother knows how to knit, ask her to show you how. If your grandfather's first language is not one you know, ask him to teach you how to say things in that language. Even something as simple as teaching you a card game or how they used to cook a special dish can remind someone that they still have skills to pass along, that someone can still benefit from their knowledge. Giving them the opportunity to pass along their knowledge and wisdom can be a gift you give them—and one from which you will benefit as well.

BREATHE TOGETHER:
A CALMING TECHNIQUE

When someone with dementia begins to get stressed, their breathing usually quickens—and that often leads to self-perpetuating anxiety. One technique that works well to break the cycle of anxiousness is to slow down the breathing; taking three slow, deep breaths and letting them out slowly—if possible, breathing in through the nose and out through the mouth, as in "yoga breathing"—can readjust the breathing pattern and help someone calm down. Say to your grandmother, "I learned a technique that could help you feel better. Do you want to try it with me? We'll take three slow, deep breaths together; follow me, do what I do." Sitting close in front of her, have her take those three slow, deep breaths along with you, as slowly as you—and she—can. Chances are, you will both find yourselves in a calmer state.

CHAPTER FIVE

HOW DOES DEMENTIA AFFECT FAMILY AND FRIENDS?

The burden of having someone with dementia in the family is more than dealing with the actual tasks involved in caregiving, whether the responsibility falls on one person or is shared, and whether there are paid helpers involved as well. There is an emotional and psychic toll on every individual in the family, as well as on the family unit as a whole. It is helpful to consider how dementia affects an entire family. Some of these are areas in which you, as a teen, might be able to help or make a difference. Others will probably be things only an adult will be able to handle. Thinking about them and recognizing how they may impact your family as a whole can help you help yourself and your family, too. What are some of the issues and behaviors that make up this burden?

RAW AND UNEXPECTED EMOTIONS CAN BE HARD

Josef described a particularly poignant scene that made a significant impact on him. Said Josef,

My grandmother—my dad's mom—was very demented when she got old. She moved into a nursing home and lived there until she was almost 100. It was sad to see how she went downhill. It got to the point where she couldn't recognize my father, her son. He would go to visit and ask,

"Do you know who I am, Mom? Who am I, Mom?" She never did, and after a while, he just stopped asking if she knew who he was. She noticed that he wasn't asking her if she knew him anymore. She would try to talk, but she couldn't really talk. One day when we visited, she tried to say my sister's name; my sister had lived with my grandmother, and they were close. Her name was Meghan, and that day, my grandmother tried to say, "Meghan." My dad just—I'd never seen my dad cry, but I saw him cry then. Wow. That really hit me.

DEMENTIA IS SOMETIMES A FAMILY SECRET

Even though there is more and more public discussion about dementia and there are many organizations and community groups that offer information and activities for people with dementia and their families, there remains, for many people, stigma about the loss of mental capacity. Some families feel strongly about keeping their medical concerns private, and some people may even feel shame that there is dementia in the family. The strain of trying to keep a secret can be a significant cause of stress in an individual or a family.

DEMENTIA'S PUBLIC FACE
CAN BE DISTURBING

It is hard to ignore some of the more blatant behaviors of someone with dementia, and when you are in public with your grandmother and she behaves strangely or inappropriately, it can be hard to know what to do and easy to feel embarrassment or even anger. Keep in mind that your grandmother cannot recognize her behaviors as being inappropriate. Take steps to deal with the situation as calmly and smoothly as you can. Are you pushing your grandmother in a wheelchair through a grocery store and someone points out that she has just unbuttoned her blouse?

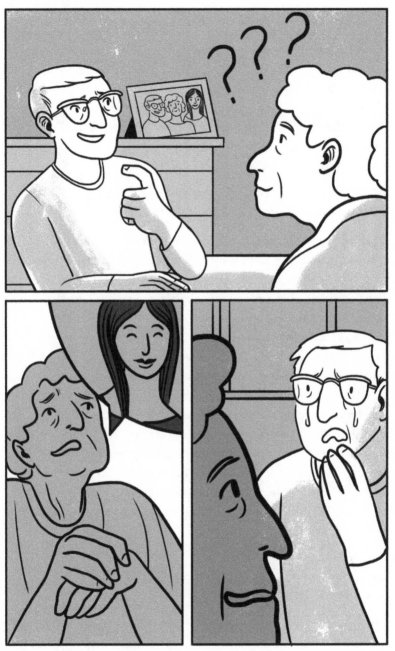

Josef's grandmother struggled to recognize her family members, but one day, when she tried to say his sister's name, they knew she still remembered them.
Illustration by Kate Haberer

Thank the person for pointing it out and see if you can calmly button her buttons. Rather than getting upset and scolding her, suggest to your grandmother that if she's too warm, you can change to lighter clothes when you get home, or that you will take her outside to cool off in a minute. Try to resolve the issue and cover her appropriately without turning the episode into a "major incident."

EMBARRASSMENT AT SOCIALLY INAPPROPRIATE BEHAVIORS (SEXUAL, VERBAL, PHYSICAL)

Dementia causes behaviors that do not conform to our social expectations. Because the person with dementia cannot help themselves prevent such behaviors, it is up to us to recognize that we cannot take them personally, but we can help explain or smooth over the disturbance they can cause.

One particularly distressing element of dementia is when the restraints that curb and formalize sexual behavior no longer hold. Someone with dementia might make sexual or lewd comments that are offensive or try to make sexual advances toward someone, whether a stranger, a helper, or even a relative. While these behaviors are disturbing, it is important to remember that the person who is making them is unable to recognize that they are inappropriate. Try to change the subject or divert their attention; make sure to keep yourself—and them—safe. Recognize that these behaviors are not directed at *you*; they are part of a disturbed and unrestrained consciousness that does not conform to our societal conventions.

WHEN SOMEONE REMOVES CLOTHING AT INAPPROPRIATE TIMES OR PLACES

It is not uncommon for someone with dementia to try and remove their clothing at a time or place that is unexpected and inappropriate; this can be cause for embarrassment on their—or your—behalf. There may be many reasons to explain such behavior. They may be feeling too hot or too cold, as dementia can affect the regulation of body temperature.[1] They may be bothered by a zipper, seam, or crease that is uncomfortable. They may have wet or soiled their clothing and may not be able to ask for help. They may be fidgeting and agitated, and remove their clothing as part of that agitation. You can try to discover if there is a physical cause for their discomfort and alleviate it, and you can gently try to help them dress or cover them. It is never helpful to yell at them, laugh at them, or shame them for behavior that they cannot control, or be ashamed on their behalf.

PARANOIA CAN AFFECT CARING RELATIONSHIPS

One common symptom of dementia is paranoia, the feeling that people are watching you, spying on you, talking about you behind your back, or taking things from you. It can be very disconcerting when your grandmother accuses you of whispering about her or tells you that her aide is stealing her clothes. However, it is often the case that, indeed, people might be talking about her behind her back: Your mother may be discussing your grandmother's needs with the aide or talking quietly with the doctor about her care. It can be hard to ensure that necessary conversations that might distress your grandmother happen outside of her hearing—and, even if they do, she may correctly sense that they *are* discussing her.

Try to sort out reality from paranoid thinking. If your grandmother accuses her aide of stealing her clothes or jewelry, try to assess if that might indeed have happened. It is unlikely but not impossible. Try to calm your grandmother's fears by assuring her that you will look into it, or find the clothing or jewelry she thinks has been stolen and show it to her. You may not be able to reassure her or erase her paranoid thinking. If she perseveres with her accusations or beliefs, the best course might be to tell her confidently that you will see if you can find out what happened and try to deflect her attention to something else.

AGGRESSIVE AND ARGUMENTATIVE BEHAVIOR ADDS TO STRESS

People with dementia sometimes become argumentative and even physically aggressive. Keep in mind that they often know that their abilities are diminishing, and it can be terribly frustrating to them to be losing independence and control in their lives, or to recognize that they are losing their memories and their ability to communicate effectively. Frustration can lead them to lash out physically, and while they may be increasingly frail, they are still able to cause damage to themselves or others. In such cases, see if you can lower the tension by speaking soothingly—*without* being condescending or infantilizing (talking to them as if they were a child), stepping away a little to give them more personal space (and to keep yourself out of harm's way), and, if possible, diverting their attention to something else.

RUDE JOKES OR COMMENTS CAN BE DISTRESSING

Making rude jokes or offensive comments in an audible tone in front of the person about whom they're speaking is not an uncommon action for someone who is demented, and that can be very uncomfortable to experience. "Look at her! She's huge!" is the type of comment you dread hearing your grandfather say when a heavyset lady is in line ahead of you at the cashier. Try not to exacerbate the situation by shushing him, accusing him of being impolite, or telling him to apologize. Try to deflect his attention to something else or move him out of proximity to that person.

ANXIETY RAISES TENSIONS

The stress of caring for someone with dementia causes concerns for everyone in the family. If the person with dementia is one of your parent's parents, keep in mind that your parent is probably feeling enormous

pressures—emotional, financial, and practical. Stress can cause people to be short-tempered, distracted, and volatile, even about nonrelated issues. Talking about it openly can be a relief and often lead to sharing ideas, suggestions, and offers of assistance that can help ease everyone's tension.

FAMILY CONVERSATIONS MAY BE PRIVATE

Some families feel that children and young adults do not need to be included in discussions or decision-making about their loved one with dementia. If that is the case in your family, it may be because they don't want to burden or distress you or feel that they need to protect you from the difficult realities of dementia. This decision not only leaves you out of a crucial part of your family's life, but also can make you feel that you are not a full participant in something important. You can take it upon yourself to open the conversation by asking questions, but I suggest that you choose an occasion when your parents have time and are not in the midst of a stressed moment. You may find that when the topic becomes open to conversation, you have valuable ideas or comments to offer.

AL'S INPUT

Al, as a young musician, spent a lot of time with his grandmother throughout her decline from Alzheimer's disease. Said Al,

> I remember how it became a topic of conversation whenever the family was together. Even when I was in my early teens, I felt that the more I knew, the more information I had, the more helpful it was in my understanding of the situation. Because music was something I was able to do with my grandmother, I felt it was a way I could be helpful. It was something I was able to contribute to her care, as well as something I could talk about with the family during those conversations. It made me feel included in an all-encompassing situation.

DEMENTIA CAN BRING
FINANCIAL BURDENS

Caring for someone with dementia can cause severe financial burdens. The cost of hiring home-care aides can be a drain on a family's finances; the cost of suitable housing can be high. For many families, these financial burdens can be crippling—and the toll they take in worry, arguments, tightened budgets, and uncertainties can be enormous. While you, as a teenager, may not be able to take an active part in easing those burdens, you can be sympathetic to them and aware that you have an impact on them as well. Be sensitive to the fact that financial burdens may necessitate changes in your economic outlook, especially when it comes to such things as getting a job, not being able to afford anything that is not a necessity, or needing to rethink where you might go to college. Recognize that such burdens are part of being a family and are a shared responsibility; keep in mind that your parents may be distressed about how such burdens will affect you. Being able to talk about them may alleviate some of the tension and even provide some new ideas about how to deal with them.

FAMILY MEMBERS HAVE
DIFFERENT PERSPECTIVES

You may find that some people in your immediate and extended family stress more about the situation, while others are more relaxed or seemingly indifferent. These differences in how they think about or deal with having a loved one with dementia can cause tensions to arise between family members. While you may not be able to solve those tensions, you *can* help by being sensitive to them, trying not to take sides, and otherwise keeping your cool.

YOUR FRIENDS MAY NOT UNDERSTAND

You may find yourself having to explain to your friends that you dropped soccer practice or can't go to the mall with them on the weekend because you're spending time with your grandfather. While some of your friends—particularly those who have loving relationships with their elders or know and enjoy your grandfather—will understand, others may not see why you spend time with someone who may not even recognize you. This can be a "teaching moment" for you to take the time to tell them what it means to you to be able to do it and what it means to your grandfather to have you there. For those who just don't get it, shrug it off and think how sad it is that they don't have the same opportunity to know and love a grandparent with dementia.

TENSIONS FLARE WHEN SOMEONE FEELS THEY BEAR MOST OF THE BURDENS

Oftentimes, whether because of geographic proximity, availability, or just personal willingness, one member of the family tends to—or seems to—undertake more of the caregiving responsibility than others. This can cause anger, frustration, resentment, and lifelong rifts in the family. Caring for someone with dementia can take a lot of time. If it is one of your parents who is bearing that burden, however willingly and lovingly, it may mean that they have to cut back on their work schedule or even give up a job. That can cause additional tensions, resentments, and financial burdens on the family. Understanding the situation will help *you* sort out what you can, although you may not be able to have any effect on it.

DISTANCE CAN FOSTER GUILT, WORRY, AND RESENTMENT

Sometimes family members live far from one another; often, that is a situation that cannot be helped, and sometimes it is a geographic expression of the family dynamic. Be aware that your parents or other family members may resent the fact that, because of geographic proximity, they may bear more of the burden of care than those who live farther away. The people who live at a distance may harbor feelings of guilt that they are not able to do more. These grudges, feelings of guilt, and resentments often are not solely due to the actual distance but may be the result of long-held, almost ancient, family dynamics.

DEMENTIA CREATES CONCERNS ABOUT LIVING ARRANGEMENTS

As dementia progresses, one of the main questions is where that person will be able to live and for how long. Will they be able to remain in their own home? When will they need more help? How will those costs be paid for? Will they need to move to a retirement community, assisted living facility, or nursing home? Will they be living with their spouse, partner, or caretaker, or an unrelated housemate?

Although it is sometimes possible for a person with dementia to remain in their own home, it can require complicated, costly, and ever-changing adjustments to be able to meet their increasing needs. Some families decide to bring their loved ones to live with them, but that, too, requires a great deal of management and adjustments, and can be a source of additional stress on family members. Possible alternative living arrangements include an assisted living facility, where there will be staff to provide some degree of support; a nursing home, when a person requires more supportive care; or a continuing care community, which offers differing levels of care, from completely independent living through assisted living, to nursing home care. Making decisions about housing and care is complicated and often emotionally stressful for the entire family.

EVERYONE WORRIES ABOUT THE FUTURE

It is natural to worry about the future and how your grandparent will decline or what it will mean to your family. Chances are, your parents are thinking about this, and so are your siblings or other close friends and family. Talking about these concerns can help you and may help others in your family understand your feelings better and possibly their own. Writing about your concerns in a journal or working out your fears creatively in a story or poem can help you sort out your worries and face them with thoughtfulness.

PEOPLE EXPERIENCE PREMATURE GRIEF AND MOURNING

You may find yourself thinking about your loved one's death and feel a great sadness in advance of it; your family is probably doing the same. Although grieving in advance can help you prepare for inevitable loss, having that grief overwhelm you can keep you from doing the practical, loving things that can be meaningful and useful in the meantime. Find a balance, if you can, between being sad about what is ahead and taking positive action in the present. Bear in mind that whatever you do for your grandparent with love, kindness, compassion, and understanding is the greatest gift that you can offer them and will be something you will hold in your heart long after they are gone.

CHAPTER SIX

ACTIVITIES TO SHARE WITH SOMEONE WITH DEMENTIA

Although just *being there* can be of tremendous importance and value for people with dementia, there are many creative, worthwhile, and even fun ways in which you can interact with them at every stage of the disease. Depending on where they are on the journey through dementia, the effectiveness and type of activities will vary. There are some things you can easily do when they are in the earlier stages of the disease and continue in varying ways as their abilities decline, and there are some activities that will begin to be less useful, effective, and sensible as their disease worsens. As the disease progresses, their concentration will diminish, their willingness or energy to engage in activities may flag, and their tolerance for activities that overwhelm their abilities may disappear. It is up to you to be sensitive to the changes in their behavior and what they will tolerate, and modify your expectations and interactions in accordance with what they are able and willing to do. If you try an activity and it seems to make your loved one anxious or frustrated, it is probably beyond their abilities and may only distress them. In that case, back off that activity and switch to something else.

Be creative, nonjudgmental, and flexible. Almost *anything* can become an activity to share; it can be a means to interact without struggling to make conversation. It also can—and should—be an opportunity to talk easily. Even if your grandmother can no longer put words together to make a sentence, she may be able to repeat words you say

> ## SOMETHING TO THINK ABOUT:
> ## CHANGE CAN BE OVERWHELMING
>
> Even the act of *changing* activities can overwhelm someone whose brain is trying hard to function; it may be wiser, if one activity makes your grandmother anxious or distressed, to sit quietly or try to have a quiet conversation instead of attempting another activity right away.

as you engage together, and she may take comfort in hearing *you* speak, even when she no longer can.

Engaging in activities is a way to share meaningful and enjoyable moments; it can also be a way to *change a mood*. If looking at old pictures makes your grandfather sad because he can no longer remember the names of the people pictured, perhaps that is a good time to ask him to tell you a story about when he was young. It might help to ask him a specific question that might raise a pleasant memory or reminiscence, for example, "Did you play baseball when you were a little boy?"

Getting involved in some activities can also be an important source of sensory stimulation. As people get older, their senses—touch, taste, smell, sight, and hearing—tend to lose their sharpness. Finding ways to engage those senses can be beneficial in reawakening memories and awareness, as well as being an enjoyable shared sensation. Some of the activities in this chapter offer ways to stimulate the senses in an enjoyable way.

As with anything else, when you are dealing with someone with dementia, always ask whether they would like to do an activity—and you don't have to name it as an "activity." When suggesting any of these activities, if you are met with any resistance, you might try to gently encourage, explain, and suggest that it is something you would enjoy doing *with* them or something you would like to teach them to do so you can do it together. Remember that they are entitled to choose *not* to do something and make choices, even if—unless it is a matter of safety—*you* think it's not the best choice.

Whether you are visiting your loved one in their own home, they are visiting you in yours, or you are visiting them in an assisted living facility or nursing home, find ways to incorporate some of these activities into your visits. You will help keep your loved one's mind and body working to the best of their abilities, and enhance the enjoyment you can both have during your visits.

SOMETHING TO THINK ABOUT: FOCUS ON ABILITIES

With any of these activities, focus on what your loved one *can* do, not what they *can't*; focus on their *ability*, not their *disability*.

While most of the activities listed below are grouped into suggestions for each stage of dementia, any of them can be modified or attempted no matter where on the dementia continuum your loved one is. It's up to you to see what works and what is enjoyable, and make whatever modifications you find work best with *your* loved one.

One important thing to remember is that no matter what their level of abilities and willingness to participate in activities, if you have a warm, affectionate relationship, or even a relationship that might not be an easy or open one, very often your simple *presence*, your willingness to be available to them, will be the most valuable—and most appreciated—thing you can offer.

OPPORTUNITIES FOR MEANINGFUL CONVERSATION

One thing that many older people feel is that they no longer have any usefulness and their life is no longer worthwhile. In the early stages of dementia, they may focus on these feelings, especially as they start to realize that their mental abilities are becoming less certain. Their days of working productively, whether at an outside job or in the home, are past. In many ways, their very identity is no longer there, especially when their most profound role, as a parent or grandparent, no longer seems to be necessary.

When these thoughts are in their minds, your grandparents may talk about their feelings; they may talk about how their life has no purpose, that they are losing their memories, or that they are afraid or sad. Although these conversations can be emotionally difficult for you to listen to, they can be an enormously meaningful connection to have with someone you love. *Honor* your grandparents' feelings and appreciate that they feel close enough to you to talk about them. Listen thoughtfully, sensitively, and empathetically. Don't feel that you must necessarily respond verbally to what they say, or try to change their outlook, or deny that there is any truth in what they say. Listen and let them know that you hear them. Rather than trying to dispute what they say or change the subject, it can be more beneficial and meaningful to you both to say something like, "It means so much to me, Gramma, that you can talk to me about these things. I don't have any answers, but I love that we can talk together like this."

Similarly, don't feel that you must necessarily change the subject if the subject is a sad one. Sometimes talking about things that are sad, such as recollections of someone who has died, is an important part of thinking about life. I remember talking with an elderly woman in the hospital who became teary when telling me about her sister, who had died. "Would you rather we talk about something else?" I asked. "Oh no," she answered, "It does me good to remember her and talk about her."

THE MAGIC OF MUSIC

I've always found it amazing to sit with someone with dementia and sing together. It is astonishing, and there are scientific explanations for this, how a person with late-stage dementia who has lost the ability to speak can suddenly summon up the words and tune of a well-known song and sing along. Something in their brain is tapped and revived by familiar music and enables them to bring forth the words and tunes residing there. As world-renowned neurologist and author Oliver Sacks wrote,

> Perhaps most remarkably, people with Alzheimer's disease and other dementias can respond to music when nothing else reaches them. Alzheimer's can totally destroy the ability to remember family members or events from one's own life—but musical memory somehow survives the ravages of disease, and even in people with advanced dementia, music can often reawaken personal memories and associations that are otherwise lost.[1]

The simplest and best-known song can be sung again and again, and bring joy and comfort to you both. Whether it is "This Land Is Your Land," "God Bless America," or "The Itsy-Bitsy Spider," singing together can be an immensely gratifying experience and a pleasure for you both. I'm certainly not a wonderful singer—sometimes it's hard for me to keep in tune—but that never matters when I'm singing with someone with diminished mental abilities; the fun of singing together, laughing if you remember—or forget, or make up—the words to a song, can be a spontaneous opportunity for pleasure and interaction, and a good way to distract someone who's beginning to become agitated or upset.

Although there are plenty of songbooks available that have the words and music for old tunes, there's no need to rely on them. You can search on your mobile phone and find the words or music to almost any song. Sometimes simple children's songs can be the easiest and most remembered; you can find lyrics, music, and animation for many songs online, and that can be an easy way to get you started. Find the song on your phone, put the phone where you both can watch, and sing along together—there are counting songs ("The Ants Go Marching Ten by Ten," "One Little, Two Little, Three Little Indians"), activity songs ("The Wheels on the Bus," "The Itsy-Bitsy Spider," "I'm a Little Teapot"), and nursery rhymes ("Mary Had a Little Lamb"), which you probably remember and may feel silly singing and gesturing to at first, but you will probably find yourself laughing along with your grandfather as you do, and it's something you can return to again and again.

Singing can be a great activity to share with someone no matter what their level of mental ability. It has no time limit, no tools are required, it needs no special skills, and it is something almost anyone can do. It can be an excellent time filler or a welcome diversion from a threatened meltdown. If there are more people around than just you and your grandmother (an aide, a friend, another visitor), encourage them to join in as well; it is one of those activities where it is truly a case of "the more, the merrier."

AL'S STORY: HOW USING MUSIC CAN DEVELOP A RELATIONSHIP

Al is a young professional music therapist, but even before he trained and became certified to do music therapy, he found that music was a way he could connect with his grandmother as her cognitive abilities declined. Said Al,

> Music was something I could do, a way I could be helpful. It was something I had to contribute, and it gave me something to talk about with the family. The basics were already there for Gramma. She never thought of herself as musical. She'd listen to classical music on the radio but was not able to carry a tune; that was something she was able to laugh about and about which we always teased her. Whenever she called us to sing happy birthday, it was hilarious. But when she started to lose her abilities, it turned out that it wasn't the music she said she loved. It was that making music with her was a way to go back to her childhood, and it was the core stuff that came out of her. Doing music with her,

singing with her, always gave us something to talk about. For Gramma, memories were what felt most comfortable for her; using music to bring back those memories turned out to be a way to communicate with her. She even surprised herself; more than once, Gramma would say, "I never knew I could remember these things, like music."

When I became a music therapist, one of the most significant things I learned about using music therapy with people with disabilities—including disabilities like Gramma had when she had Alzheimer's, is that when everything else in their lives is about disability, doing music and music therapy is about ability. With Gramma, doing music with her was playful, fun, and empowering. It was activating neural pathways; those pathways in her brain that were deteriorating due to her disease were being activated through music.

When we first began doing music together, it was very interactive; Gramma was remembering songs from her childhood, we were talking about the memories that those songs brought back, and it gave me a whole repertoire of info. As she declined, doing music together became more repetitive—so repetitive. I must have sung "Bicycle Built for Two" and "Goodnight, Irene" so many times. But these were the songs that were able to give her some pleasure, some connection, and even soothed her. To me, it was the most important thing—the thing I could give her.

ACTIVITIES FOR EARLY-STAGE DEMENTIA

PLAY CARD GAMES

If your grandparent was a card player, try to engage them in a game that they played in the past, such as gin rummy or hearts. If not, you might try one of the simple children's card games like Go Fish or Uno and see whether they can be enjoyable to play together.

PLAY CONCENTRATION

Concentration, another table game, was an entertaining memory game we used to play when we were young and can be enjoyable to do with someone who is still able to retain some short-term memory. Collect a bunch of varied objects, place them on a tray, cover them with a cloth or lid to hide them from view, lift the cover for a brief amount of time, cover them again, and try to recall the objects. For someone in early-stage dementia, try using five to ten familiar objects from around the house and see whether your grandmother can remember even a couple of them when you play. If not, the game is probably beyond her abilities at that stage, and—unless she seems to enjoy it and not be frustrated by it—you should probably avoid playing it.

PLAY BOARD GAMES

If it's an early stage of mental decline, a more complicated board game like Scrabble or Monopoly may still be possible. If those games are too complicated, it might be worth stepping back and trying a simpler game like Chutes and Ladders. It is important, however, to be sensitive to frustration or confusion and not worry about sticking to the rules if it still seems to be an enjoyable activity.

LOOK AT PHOTOS TOGETHER, MAKE A PHOTO ALBUM, OR START A SCRAPBOOK

Photos can be an enormous source of pleasure, reminiscence, story-telling, and sharing personal history. If your grandfather has framed pictures in the room, ask him to tell you about them. If you know who is in the photo but he no longer remembers, tell him whatever you can about the picture, the people in it, or the place where it was taken. Look at photo albums or help sort and organize loose photos into albums or scrapbooks. Consider jotting down information about the photos on the back—your grandfather may be the only person left who can identify people or places in the pictures, and if he is no longer able to remember, flipping the photo over to read what is written on the back can help memories resurface for him. This can be an opportunity for storytelling, memory recollection, or just conversation.

LOOK AT MAGAZINES TOGETHER

You can read aloud or look at pictures and talk about what you see. Judge your grandparent's ability to read and understand, and also see what their interests are.

DRAW, PAINT, OR SCULPT TOGETHER

Whether or not your grandparent has had any experience drawing or painting in the past, it is often surprising what putting crayons or a paintbrush into someone's hand can bring out. Using simple art materials such as crayons, colored pencils, or watercolor paints together can sometimes produce an unexpected sense of freedom and creativity, and it is also a good activity to spark conversation at almost any level. Talking about colors, textures, and images can offer a world of possibility; when there is no right or wrong, no technique to be followed, you both have the chance to relax and have fun together. Just encourage enjoyment of the moment and the freedom to express feelings or thoughts on paper. Similarly, and especially for older people who have issues like arthritis that may make holding a pencil or paintbrush difficult, using soft children's' modeling clay to create figures, familiar objects, or simply abstract forms offers a creative outlet, and the act of manipulating clay is also a good hand exercise that can help ease stiffness and promote flexibility.

BRING A FRIEND TO VISIT

Sometimes bringing a friend with you can help make a visit more entertaining for both you and your grandparent, as it doubles the conversational possibilities. If your friend does not know what to expect of your grandmother's abilities or behavior, explain it as helpfully as you can so that your friend will be comfortable and know how to respond. If your friend is someone your grandmother has met before, remind her of when they met or whom they might know in common. Talk about how you became friends or what you like to do together. Keep in mind that when someone has dementia, it may be difficult to process two people talking at once, so try not to talk over one another or at the same time.

PLAY THE MIRROR GAME OR "MIRRORING"

Mirroring is a fun—and fascinating—way to communicate with someone nonverbally. It has a remarkable power to connect two people without words and be genuinely "in the moment" with someone. It is an especially useful tool to use with someone who has trouble connecting with the outside world. When you *do* get into it, you may find it amazing how in sync you are with your loved one.

Mirroring is simple. Sit face-to-face with the other person, making sure you are both comfortable and close enough to touch. Look into one another's eyes. As you maintain eye contact throughout the exercise, mirror whatever movements your partner makes. Try to keep movements slow and match your breathing to your partner's breaths. The goal is for you to *actively* listen and watch, and feel what your partner is feeling—to be "in the moment" with them. If they move their hand, you move your hand—as simultaneously and identically as you can—without giving up the eye contact. Take your cues from your partner; if they move slowly, you move slowly; if they speed up, you speed up. Chances are, after a few minutes, you will feel a very powerful, nonverbal connection.

MAKE CONVERSATION

Sometimes making conversation with someone with dementia can be more of a monologue than a dialogue. As thinking, concentration, and even speech become more difficult for them, they might still appreciate and want the pleasure of hearing someone speak to them. In that circumstance, the burden is more on you to keep up *your* end of the conversation. How do you do that?

Tell your grandmother about your day, your friends, your hobbies, and your fears or dreams; it doesn't matter if she can't understand or isn't able to participate in a conversation—hearing your voice, enjoying just having you there, and having you talk to her can give her pleasure and comfort. As you become more comfortable speaking your thoughts aloud, you will probably find that it becomes easier. If you want a loving, nonjudgmental sounding board in whom you can confide things you might not tell anyone else, pouring your heart out to a beloved grandparent who can no longer speak can be a wonderful relief.

ENCOURAGE "LIFE REVIEW" OR REMINISCENCE

Many gerontologists (people who study the field of aging) and geriatricians (medical doctors who specialize in older people) believe that "life review," or recalling and thinking about the events and course of one's life, is a crucial part of what they consider "successful aging." Being able to think about what you did in life, the people in your life, what you enjoyed doing, and perhaps what you wish you had done differently are all part of life review. You can provide an opportunity for your grandparents to engage in life review by asking them to tell you stories from their past. Ask them to tell you stories about their childhood, families, young adulthood, early days as a parent, and favorite things or activities from the past. Some questions that can get reminiscences started are as follows:

- Did you have a favorite dress or pair of shoes?

- How did you meet Grandpa (Grandma)?

- What did you do for fun?

- What were your favorite foods?

- How/when did you learn English?

- Did you celebrate your birthdays as a child?

ACTIVITIES FOR MID-STAGE DEMENTIA

EAT TOGETHER

Throughout human history, eating has been a social activity. Although you might occasionally enjoy eating by yourself, eating with family or friends can greatly enhance the experience. For people with moderate dementia, eating tends to become less enjoyable. Oftentimes, the sense of taste becomes less acute, which can affect the pleasure of eating. Meals can be more challenging to manage; the texture of foods may become discomforting; and, with the feeling of isolation and loneliness that often accompanies dementia, it just may not be tempting for them to eat. Maintaining adequate nutrition and hydration becomes more difficult.

You can help by sharing a meal; having a cup of tea together; or otherwise joining your loved one to make this a more entertaining, social, and pleasurable time. Even if you don't eat an entire meal with them (your meal schedule may be very different than theirs), sit with them and have something to drink or a snack, and chat while they eat. If their appetite seems to falter, find ways to urge them to eat and drink, even a little bit at a time. Your friendly encouragement and participation may make the difference in their eating and not eating, or not eating (or drinking) enough.

ENGAGE IN PUPPETRY

If you have hand puppets or finger puppets, or if you are creatively inclined and would like to make puppets on your own, using puppets to encourage interaction and conversation can be a fun and laughter-provoking game for you and your grandparent. Put a puppet on your hand and another on your grandmother's hand, and have them talk to one another; you might ask your grandmother to tell her about her puppet. Does she have a name? Where was she born? Does she like to eat birthday cake? Any story line that you make up—or, better yet, make up together—can bring out words, memories, and laughter—all good things for someone with memory issues.

PARTICIPATE IN PHYSICAL ACTIVITIES

Take a Walk

If your loved one can walk, whether on her own or with an assistive device like a cane, walker, or rollator, taking a walk with them is both a healthy physical activity and a way to visit and interact. Turn the walk into a wonderfully interactive experience. A walk outdoors, on the street, or in a park can be an opportunity to talk, point things out, make conversation about what you see, or explore memories. A walk through a store can be an opportunity to point out familiar items, ask about memories ("Who washed your hair when you were a little girl, Gramma?"), or talk about colors or sizes. Even a walk in a hallway can be a time for conversation ("Should we go to the next doorway, Grampa? How many steps should we take?). Point out things of interest or something you know they appreciated in the past.

My mother always had a love of babies, and even when she was no longer able to speak, seeing a baby always brought a smile to her face. We would sit on a bench in front of her building, and when a mother passed by with a small baby in a stroller, I would point out the baby and often the mother happily brought the baby close, and my mother would wave or waggle her fingers, and try to engage with the baby—and when the baby smiled or stretched out a little hand, my mother responded happily. Even with toddlers or young children, their mothers would often bring them close and use it as an opportunity to teach their little ones social engagement and the joys of interacting with a frail, older person. As with every other activity, when dealing with someone with dementia, modulate your pace and level to theirs, and be sensitive to when they might have had enough.

Do Household Tasks

Do simple household tasks together, for example, folding laundry; take a warm bundle of towels out of the dryer and spread them on your laps or a table. Work together to fold the towels and stack them in a pile. It is probably an activity for which your grandmother has motor memory, something physical that she has done so many times before that her muscles remember it automatically, without thinking. If your grandmother is not able to fold towels, just handling the warm, soft cloth and moving her fingers over it while you talk gently with her can be a soothing and pleasurable activity to do together.

If your grandmother enjoyed cooking, even if she is no longer able to do it herself, you can still help her reenact familiar routines. Whether it is something as simple as letting her put her teabag into a cup of hot water or giving her a wooden spoon and mixing bowl to help you by stirring batter, engaging her in familiar routines can be entertaining and comforting.

USE A MYSTERY GRAB BAG

In a paper, plastic, or cloth bag, place several familiar, small, common objects; have your grandmother reach into the bag without looking and pull out an object; see if she can name the object and talk about how it can be used. If she can't identify or talk about an object, help her by naming it and talking about it. The following are some everyday objects you might include. Use your imagination and creativity to think of others.

- Clean, dry sponge
- Bottle or can opener
- Small kitchen strainer
- Coin purse with several coins in it
- Small stuffed animal or doll
- Little toy or ball
- Key

- Pair of sunglasses

- Lipstick or makeup compact

- Pen, pencil, and eraser

- Pincushion (remove the pins first!)

- Glove

- Wooden spoon

- Small hairbrush, comb, or nailbrush

READ POETRY ALOUD

For many of the same reasons that music and song lyrics provide pleasurable feelings and links to memories, so does poetry. Both forms incorporate rhythm and repetition, and, when well-known or familiar, a comforting sense of control. Try reading poems that have a strong sense of rhythm and repeated phrases or present a strong sense of setting or scene. Some good choices for reading aloud include the following:

- "The Raven" by Edgar Allen Poe

- "Annabel Lee" by Edgar Allen Poe

- "The Road Not Taken" by Robert Frost

- "Stopping by Woods on a Snowy Evening" by Robert Frost

- "The Highwayman" by Alfred Noyes

- "The Owl and the Pussycat" by Edward Lear

- "Jabberwocky" by Lewis Carroll

- "Casey at the Bat" by Ernest Lawrence Thayer

- "The Land of Counterpane" by Robert Louis Stevenson

ENGAGE IN SIMPLE PHYSICAL EXERCISES

As dementia settles in, people tend to become less mobile and more sedentary. Finding ways to keep their body moving helps keep joints and muscles from becoming stiff from disuse. Whether it's fingers, hands, feet, toes, or face, there are simple exercises that almost anyone can do until very late stages of dementia. Be sensitive to your grandfather's physical abilities; muscles and joints may be stiff, and arthritis can cause joint pain and stiffness as well. These simple exercises can be done sitting in a chair, and most can even be done lying in bed. Engage your grandmother in following your simple motions; by turning them into a game, something you do together—laughing, joking, and even being silly about it—you can help an older person with dementia stay engaged and moving, even for short periods of time. Make these exercises interactive by having them follow your motions.

Simple Hand Exercises

Remember "Open/Shut Them" from nursery school? Sit facing your grandmother and do the following: Open your hands wide, then shut them into fists, and repeat. Making a fist, raise each finger as if counting on your hand, and repeat or do the reverse from an open hand to closed fist by lowering each finger. With palms on your knees, raise just the fingers and tap them down and repeat.

Simple Foot Exercises

With feet flat on the floor, raise the heels and lower them, and repeat. With feet flat on the floor, raise the toes and lower them, and repeat. Starting with feet flat on the floor, march your legs up and down, alternating left and right.

Facial Exercises

Open your eyes as wide as you can. Open your mouth in a big "O." Move your jaw side to side. Stick out your tongue as far as you can.

Exercises with Koosh Balls, Stress Balls, and Bead Balls

Whether they are toys or physical therapy tools, there are many types of flexible spheres or squishy, bead-stuffed animals that are great for exercising fingers and hands, and encouraging different sensory experiences.

Balloon Activities

Blow up a balloon and toss it back and forth; this is both a game and an exercise that encourages eye–hand coordination and reflexes.

Bubble Activities

If you have or can purchase an inexpensive bottle of children's bubble liquid and wand, blowing bubbles—together if your grandmother is able or for her if she is not—can provide a fun, interactive, and motivating experience. Reaching to poke bubbles, admiring them, and laughing when they break can be something you share. It can also help spark memories of childhood and conversation about them.

SOMETHING TO THINK ABOUT: HELPING WITH THERAPEUTIC ACTIVITIES

If your grandparent is working with a physical or occupational therapist, find out if they left a list or printout of exercises or therapeutic objects to use. Follow their directions and do the exercises with your grandparent. The exercise instructions are generally straightforward and easy to follow.

GARDEN

Gardening—whether indoors or out—can be a source of great pleasure and sensory stimulation. When gardening together, you can not only engage the hands but also bring in the sense of smell, as well as talk about different colors, textures, sizes, similarities, and differences, and what memories might be stirred. Even if you have no outdoor area, you can share the pleasures of planting and tending plants in indoor pots. If your grandmother has potted plants and can stand and walk around, help her water them, prune fading leaves or flowers, or even repot them if needed. If there are vases of fresh flowers, help her decide if they need more water or fresh water. If she's not able to get around, bring small plants to her and talk about them—about whether they need water or are growing or blooming. This is not only an opportunity for conversation and interaction, but also may be a way to bring back a pleasurable activity or experience that once involved her regularly. You can make the conversation more meaningful by bringing in *her* importance and usefulness in helping to keep the plants healthy, thereby reinforcing that your grandmother has a purpose and value in daily life.

PLAY TABLE GAMES

Table games like Dominoes, Connect Four, and Jenga can be enjoyable to play together and are also a good way to help an older person with hand and finger exercise and coordination. They can also provide mental activity and social engagement. Don't feel as if you need to stick to the rules, especially if your grandfather's memory won't let him keep to them. It's easy to make up other ways to play with the pieces, especially if you are flexible and creative. Can't keep score for Dominoes? See if you can count the dots together and look for another piece with the same number. Similarly, with Uno or other card games, connect numbers, colors, and shapes; there are many ways to use the tiles, cards, or pieces to interact and play.

GIVE A MANICURE

Doing a gentle manicure, especially if it includes a hand massage with a nicely scented lotion, can be a lovely way to share a sensory experience with someone. Even picking a color of polish can turn into fun. Naming colors, comparing them, and asking which one is the favorite choice bring about conversation, laughter, and the mental activity of naming colors or making choices. Be careful, however, if you are filing nails, to avoid any discomfort; be sensitive as to whether this may be an uncomfortable sensation for your elder.

ACTIVITIES FOR LATE-STAGE DEMENTIA

SOMETHING TO THINK ABOUT: TOUCH

As people age, along with the losses they face in their diminishing abilities, they also often lose the pleasure of experiencing human touch. They may no longer routinely hold hands with a loved one; they may no longer receive the casual hugs or kisses that are, for many people, a part of daily life. Touch is an essential human sensation, and finding ways to share it with someone with dementia can be a soothing and wonderful experience. Be sensitive to when touch is welcome and appropriate, and when it could cause discomfort. Sitting next to your grandmother and holding her hand, stroking her arm, or giving her an extra hug or two—*if* she does not seem to mind that physical touch—can be a comfort and delight for you both.

RUB LOTION ON ARMS, LEGS, HANDS, OR FEET

Older people's skin becomes thinner, drier, and more fragile with age. Keeping it moisturized can be important in helping reduce tears in the skin and keeping it supple, especially in drier winter months. If you are comfortable doing this, suggest to your grandparent that you gently massage lotion into their skin. Some people enjoy that experience, while others may find it too intimate; again, use your sensitivity about whether this is something you would both enjoy.

COMB OR STYLE HAIR

Again, offering to comb or style hair can be a shared and comforting sensory experience. Just be sure to be gentle and keep your motions smooth and slow so as not to cause pulling, discomfort, or agitation. Keep up a conversation or find something to laugh about, as shared silliness can be a wonderful interaction.

SOMETHING TO THINK ABOUT: REFLECTING ON REFLECTIONS

It can be disconcerting for an older person with dementia to see themselves reflected in a mirror. They may not recognize the person they see, and they may not believe that the person reflected is them. Be sensitive to that; if it seems to upset your grandfather to look in the mirror, distract him and move the mirror away, or move him away from the mirror. Have you ever been startled to catch sight of yourself in a mirror or storefront unexpectedly and realize you look messier, shorter, or older than you thought? *You* can readjust your mental image—but someone with dementia may not be able to do that. Keep in mind that no matter what a person's age, oftentimes the image we have of ourselves in our mind's eye may not be what others see.

HAVE ANIMAL VISITS

There is a relatively new and specialized field called pet-assisted therapy, which uses trained and certified teams consisting of a pet and an owner or handler who bring their animals to hospitals, schools, libraries, nursing homes, and other institutions to provide comfort, support, and a nonjudgmental and gentle presence. Any well-behaved pet can be brought for a visit to a private home if animals are welcome and if you have permission to do so. (Some nursing homes will allow you to bring in a pet to visit your relative if you have documentation of up-to-date vaccinations.) If your grandparent always enjoyed animals or always had pets of their own, it can be an easy and enjoyable experience to bring your pet. They can sit on your grandmother's lap or at her feet and be petted, talked to, and talked about. It is a shared experience, a topic of conversation, and a comforting and relaxing experience.

If your loved one is not familiar or comfortable with animals, it can take some advance work—asking whether they would like to meet your pet, showing them a picture or video, talking about how gentle they are or how soft their fur is and how much they love being petted (if that is true). If you have their agreement, start with a short introductory visit; let them try to pet the animal while you hold it and see how the experience goes. From there, you might find you are making regular visits, and even when someone is no longer able to speak or engage in other activities, having a warm, soft pet in their lap or their hand lifted onto soft and warm fur can still be a comforting, pleasurable sensory experience.

JOSEF'S STORY

Josef, a young man who volunteers in a nursing home, told a story about how one lady in the memory care unit responded to the resident bird. Said Josef,

> The nursing home where I work has a lot of bird cages in various places in the buildings. Most of the birds are small and brightly colored, and the residents love to watch them. But there was this one bird, a big white bird, she lives alone in a cage near some other birds, and she talks. Most of the time, you can't understand the words she says, but there's one word she knows: "Papa." She doesn't just say it, she yells

it. One time, I brought this lady from the memory care unit down in her wheelchair. She could hardly speak, and she just kind of sat still in her wheelchair, not being responsive to anything; she just always looked blank. I was going to take her outside to the terrace, but we passed by this bird in her birdcage and stayed there for about five minutes. I could see that the lady kept trying to talk to the bird and waving at her. Finally, we had to leave, and just as I was wheeling her away, the bird started screaming, "Papa! Papa!" The lady turned around quickly. She got so excited, her eyes lit up, and all she could do was smile. I can't forget how that bird was able to get such a happy reaction from her.

Watching fish—whether in a simple goldfish bowl or a fully equipped aquarium—can be both a soothing and engaging activity. The fish do not even have to be real—it is now possible to get aquariums with artificial fish that simulate a lifelike underwater environment, which can be as entrancing as watching living fish.

There are even robotic cats and dogs that look realistic and purr or cuddle realistically in response to petting. Many nursing homes now use these mechanical pets to help soothe and comfort residents with dementia.

THE END RESULT: WHAT YOU GIVE, AND WHAT YOU TAKE AWAY

No matter how you engage with someone with dementia and no matter the stage their disease is in, being with them, sharing the present moment with them, and interacting in whatever verbal or nonverbal way gives them comfort, you will find that you take away feelings of satisfaction and accomplishment for what you can give of yourself. The dementia path is a hard one, and you will experience deeply emotional moments along the way. But when you open your heart to the journey your loved one is on and join them along the way, you will carry with you the knowledge that you gave them the gift of yourself, and you will be able to face the future with no regrets about the past.

PART III

WHAT'S NEXT

CHAPTER SEVEN

FACING DEATH AND THE RITUALS OF DEATH AND MOURNING

Her death was a loss but not a tragedy.
—author's older brother

People die. We will all die someday. We rarely know when people will die, although we sometimes know what will probably cause their death and perhaps even how they will likely die. For many years, it was thought that people did not die *of* dementia, that while people may die *with* dementia, it would be something else that would ultimately be the cause of death. In recent years, however, that thinking has changed. As reported in a paper published in the *New England Journal of Medicine*, "Dementia is a leading cause of death in the United States but is under-recognized as a terminal illness."[1] As *Time* magazine further explained in an article about that same paper,

> Dementia is most often thought of as a memory disorder, an illness of the aging mind. In its initial stages, that's true—memory loss is an early hallmark of dementia. But experts in the field say dementia is more accurately defined as fatal brain failure: a terminal disease, like cancer, that physically kills patients, not simply a mental ailment that accompanies older age.[2]

In an earlier chapter, I describe what to expect as death approaches. That pertains to the physical manifestations of the dying process and some of the means we can incorporate to help keep a dying person as comfortable and peaceful as possible. What I did not talk about is how this approaching death will affect you, your family, and close friends.

COMMUNICATION

Talking about death, impending death, the realities of the dying process, and what will take place after death is, for many families, a taboo subject. People may refuse to discuss these things due to a sense of denial; if they don't talk about it, it won't happen. There may be some cultural or superstitious beliefs that talking about something will affect it's happening, that talking about death may bring it on or hasten it.

The truth of the matter is that, for many people, talking openly about the impending death and everything that it will mean can be enormously comforting and help bring a family's concerns, fears, and emotions into focus. Not having to bottle up and hide fears or emotions, sharing feelings, and asking and answering questions honestly can alleviate much of the stress that is a huge part of caring for someone with dementia.

If your parent tries to have a conversation with you about what to expect, don't shy away from it. Let them know what is on your mind; you may find that talking through these difficult things brings you closer or helps you better understand and empathize with your own parent's feelings and concerns.

Speak up with sensitivity about your concerns. Perhaps you feel that your grandmother's aide is not taking as much care in feeding her as you think she should. Maybe your grandmother told you, in one of your conversations, about how she hopes her death or funeral will happen. If you want to know more about your grandmother's condition or what the expectations are for her care, voice your questions, and try to keep the avenues of conversation open as the situation progresses.

Just try to speak thoughtfully and with consideration; don't choose especially stressed moments or times when your parent's time or attention is focused on something more urgent.

WHEN YOUR LOVED ONE TALKS ABOUT DEATH

As many people get older, they become, in some sense, less afraid of dying. The older one gets, the more familiar death becomes. Friends die, loved ones die, we learn of old classmates' deaths, we attend more funerals, and we think more about our own end.

When people recognize that they are in the early stages of dementia, sometimes their thoughts turn to their decline, and ultimate death. It is not uncommon for them to voice those thoughts, and if they do, it is important and valuable to listen to them and learn more about what is on their mind. Try to resist the urge to deflect the conversation, brush it off, or change the subject to something else. Allow them to talk about their thoughts on death and dying, on how they might want their death handled. Your grandfather may have definite ideas about who he might like to speak at his funeral, whether he wants to be cremated or buried, or music to be played on that day. You can honor him by listening and helping to fulfill his wishes.

HOSPICE CARE

Hospice is a model of care focused on supporting the physical, emotional, and spiritual needs of an individual and their family during the last months of life. Hospice care in the United States is based on the hospice insurance benefit, which, for most people, can be accessed through their private medical insurance, Medicare, or Medicaid. While it can take place in a hospital or special hospice residence, most hospice care is delivered in the patient's own home, enabling many hospice patients to die peacefully at home.

A person can usually be enrolled in hospice when their physician or medical professional certifies that they are not expected to live more than six months and will no longer receive treatment for the terminal condition that is expected to cause their death. Some people do live beyond that six-month expectation and can be recertified for the hospice benefit, while others experience some improvement in their situation, reducing the need for hospice involvement. In those cases, the hospice benefit can be interrupted and reestablished later if needed.

What hospice can provide is a great deal of support and comfort for both the patient and the family. A hospice doctor can oversee care and prescribe pain medications or medications to alleviate other symptoms. A nurse will make regular visits, evaluating the status and comfort of the patient, and implementing whatever is necessary to maximize the patient's comfort. With the help of the hospice nurse, patients can receive some basic medical supplies, assistive devices, and medical equipment, depending on their needs. The nurse will evaluate their changing needs and make sure they receive whatever will be most helpful in maintaining their comfort. The nurse will also ensure that the aide or the family caregiver(s) understand what to expect and are trained in any daily medical care that might be necessary. Hospice can provide a home aide to help in personal care and a social worker to help address the emotional or social needs of the patient and family. Chaplains are usually part of the hospice team; hospice chaplains are trained in interfaith beliefs and practices, and prepared to address the spiritual needs of the patient and family following whatever their beliefs or nonbeliefs may be. Volunteers, physical and occupational therapists, and speech and language therapists will most likely also be part of the team. Grief counselors will be available to counsel family members both before and for some time after the death.

THE FINAL STAGES OF THE DYING PROCESS AND BEDSIDE VIGILS

When a person with dementia reaches the end of their life, the final stages usually include the inability to take in food or fluids, increasing immobility, and reduced responsiveness; this period of nearing death can last about three weeks. The final stage, which is called "active dying," usually takes place during the last three days of life. There are several signs that indicate death is near. These include irregular breathing, often with long pauses between breaths; unresponsiveness; decrease in urine production; agitation or fitfulness; very low blood pressure; cooling of the skin on the arms and lower legs; and, with the inability to swallow, a buildup of secretions that can cause a gurgling sound in the throat. Every effort should be taken during this time to keep the dying person calm and comfortable.

Many people choose to remain at the bedside of a dying person, known as keeping a "bedside vigil." Some cultures believe that it is important not to let a person die alone. Sitting by the side of someone you love while they leave their life behind can be a profoundly moving time for you and one you will never forget or regret; it is the ultimate gift you can give a loved one. Families may sit together or take turns staying by the bedside. You might hold your loved one's hand or simply lay your hand atop their arm; that physical connection can be soothing to you both. You might use a soft cloth to wipe their face, hands, and feet with lukewarm water. You might choose to read, nap, pray, play soft music, or just sit quietly. Whatever you do, the most important element is that you are there for your loved one.

The sense of hearing is thought to be the last of the senses to be lost. For that reason many people suggest that it is important to talk quietly to the person who is dying; to speak words of love, forgiveness, and assurance that all will be well; that you and the family will take care of one another; and that they no longer need to worry and are free to leave without regret.

Many people believe that the dying can take in these words and that such words offer comfort and, in a sense, give a person permission to die.

One thing that can occur and be particularly distressing to someone who has spent long hours at the bedside of a loved one who is dying is that when they step out of the room for a brief moment, their loved one dies. Some people believe that a dying person may hold on to life until their loved one is absent, to spare them the distress of witnessing their death. I had heard this described many times and experienced it for myself. I stayed very near my mother during the night she was dying, only leaving her side when her loving aide came to sit with her so I could shower. In those few moments, my mother died.

There are many different cultural practices concerning the last moments of life. Some people open a window in the room where a person is dying to allow their soul to leave. Catholic tradition is to have a priest present to perform the sacrament known as the Last Rites. Jewish tradition is to read from the Psalms or quietly recite or chant prayers, and to always have someone with the dying person. Some people believe that you should allow the dying person some moments alone to have peace and quiet for short periods without people around them. Whatever the customs or beliefs, the bedside vigil is a singularly profound and deeply respectful time.

WHAT HAPPENS AFTER A PERSON DIES?

I will not address the many spiritual beliefs about what happens after death; that is a subject you may explore on your own. But death also involves practical, straightforward decisions and actions that are worth knowing about. The more you know and consider, the better prepared you will be when the inevitable moment occurs. While I cannot cover the myriad decisions and actions that will take place, I will touch on some of the basic areas.

If the death occurs in a hospital or nursing home, a doctor will certify the moment of death so an official death certificate can be issued. If the death occurs at home and the patient has been in hospice care, a call to the hospice team will enable them to assist the family in taking care of the next steps. If the death occurred at home and the person who died was not in hospice care, in most cases, it is necessary to call 911. Usually, a family member or other caregiver will close the eyes of the person who died and cover them neatly with a sheet as soon as the death has been acknowledged.

DNR, POLST, AND MOLST DOCUMENTS, AND WHY THEY ARE SO IMPORTANT

DNR (Do Not Resuscitate), POLST (Physician's Orders for Life-Sustaining Treatment), or MOLST (Medical Orders for Life-Sustaining Treatment) are forms prepared with a medical professional while a person is alive. The forms spell out the wishes concerning end-of-life decisions and measures wanted—or not wanted—taken if they were not able to speak for themselves. Primary among those choices is whether they would want resuscitation attempted if their breathing or heart has stopped. An attempt to resuscitate is a physically violent and disturbing procedure, and is even more so on the frail body of a person with end-stage dementia whose heart or breathing has already stopped. Emergency personnel are required to attempt resuscitation if there is no DNR (or POLST or MOLST) indicating that resuscitation is not wanted. For this reason, it is important to have a DNR, POLST, or MOLST (state requirements differ) on hand when a person is terminally ill. Many health professionals suggest posting a copy of such a document on the refrigerator where it is easily seen and accessible.

COLLECTING THE BODY

Many families, knowing that their loved one has a terminal condition, make advance arrangements with a funeral home. If that is the case, a call made to the funeral home will activate the arrangements. Even if arrangements were not made in advance, funeral homes are usually able to handle things quickly.

Whether the body is at home, in a hospital, or at a nursing facility, the funeral home will usually dispatch two or three people to collect it; sometimes, a single person can handle it alone. Professional funeral home personnel are almost always quiet, respectful, and deliberate in what they do. They will probably ask the family members to step out of the room while they wrap the body in a zippered body bag, place it on a stretcher, and wheel it away to a waiting hearse or station wagon. Funeral personnel try to be as discrete as possible and understand that this is a time of grief and shock for those present.

FUNERAL CUSTOMS

There are many different traditions, customs, and practices as to what happens to the body after death. Some faith traditions require in-ground (or sometimes aboveground) burial or interment. Jewish and Muslim tradition requires that a funeral be held quickly, within twenty-four hours of death, or as soon after that as possible. Some religions, such as Hinduism, practice cremation (burning the body using high heat to reduce it to ashes) rather than burial; nowadays, many non-Hindu people choose cremation as well. Hindus usually hold a cremation ceremony within a day or two after death. Catholic and Christian funerals are usually held several days or a week after death. Funerals may be religious or secular (nonreligious). They may take place in a church, in a private home, in a funeral home, or at the gravesite. In some traditions, visiting with the family is done before the funeral, as in Catholic or Christian visitation hours or "wakes." Visiting with Jewish mourners may take the form of a brief greeting immediately before the funeral service begins but generally continues during a week of formal mourning in the home of the deceased or their closest family, known as "sitting Shiva." In Islamic and Hindu cultures, it is also customary for friends to visit the home of the mourners after the funeral. It is an almost universal tradition to treat the body with respect and care, formalize the process of mourning the death, and visit with the mourners to console them and offer them support.

EULOGIES: HONORING THE DEAD

In many traditions, it is the custom for close relatives or friends to make a speech at the funeral; these are generally called *eulogies*. When you and your family are discussing funeral plans, you will learn whether eulogies will be part of the service. If so, you may be asked or feel that you would like to speak about the person you lost. If everyone agrees, then this is the moment when you should sit down, organize your thoughts, decide what are the most meaningful things you might say, and *write them down*. When giving a eulogy, one should never include negative comments or speak ill of the dead. It is the time to talk of the things you loved about them, things they taught you, things you may have wished you had said, and what this person meant to you. A funny story that might even make people laugh can be an appropriate and welcome part of your speech, as long as it is loving and not something that would have embarrassed the person in life. The important thing is to gather your thoughts and words, and *write them down* and even practice them aloud, whether in privacy or to your family, in advance of the funeral. It is never a good thing to try to speak extemporaneously, without notes, particularly at a funeral. This is no time for wandering, long-drawn-out, disorganized words. Keep it short; keep it meaningful; keep it loving.

TREATMENT OF THE BODY

There are differing customs when it comes to the treatment of the body. Some people choose to embalm the body (prepare it with a preservative fluid to prevent decay) before burial. Some traditions do not allow embalming. In cases where the body has been embalmed, it may also be dressed in a carefully selected outfit and groomed to present a serene and lifelike appearance for mourners to view during visitation hours or wakes held at the funeral home. Islamic and Jewish custom calls for ritually washing the body and wrapping it in a shroud. In some cultures, the body may be buried with items that were meaningful to the person who died. Many people choose to bury their loved one in as elaborate and beautiful a coffin as they can afford, and have the coffin placed into a watertight vault to prevent decay after burial. On the other hand, the Jewish tradition is to bury a person in a simple and unadorned pine coffin, to allow for the natural disintegration of the remains.

When the choice has been to cremate the body, the ashes will be returned to the family unless other arrangements have been made. Some people choose to keep the ashes in a special urn; sometimes, the ashes are buried or placed in a *columbarium*, an area within a cemetery with niches for urns of ashes. Some families choose to sprinkle the ashes in a place that held special memories for the person who died; in that event, it is crucial to find out whether it is permissible to sprinkle ashes there. Whatever arrangements are made, it is important to treat the body or the remains with respect, acknowledging them as the final remnants of human life.

BEREAVEMENT AND MOURNING

In the days and weeks following the death, you are likely to experience many different emotions. Sadness and loss will almost certainly be high on the list of things you are feeling, especially if you had a warm and loving relationship with the person who died. You may also feel anxious about how your family is dealing with the loss or how it will change the family dynamic, as well as feeling sadness for *their* loss. You may feel guilty thinking perhaps that you did not do everything you could or should have, or maybe even because you had wished for the death to occur, as the life of your loved one seemed hopeless and unbearable. You may feel resentment at having plans derailed or jealousy at the attention paid to other members of your family. You may feel confused, exhausted, and overwhelmed by the whirl of activity that usually surrounds a death.

The period of mourning, whether a formalized ritual or an unlabeled, informal phase, can also be a time of heightened family closeness as you pay attention to one another's feelings and share in the loss. To your surprise, you may also find it can be a time of great joy and riotous laughter; reminiscing with friends and family about the person who died, retelling family stories and laughing about them, provides a welcome release from grief, a lifting of the family stresses that may have preceded the death, and a way to celebrate the life that was lived. The days or weeks of mourning after a death often bring distant family members or old friends together and enable opportunities to rekindle affection and grow closer to people you don't see often. It is a time for people to reconnect and remember why family and community are so important in our lives.

When the person who died experienced years of cognitive decline, it is not uncommon to feel that, in a sense, you lost them long before their life ended. Oftentimes, because the progress of dementia can be so heartrending—even excruciating—to watch, death comes as something of a relief. You may feel guilty, in fact, at feeling relief; but hopefully you can take comfort in reviewing the good years of the person's life, the enjoyment you shared, and the knowledge that you were able to give them your love, attention, and presence when it mattered the most.

While the death of a person with dementia can be a time of sadness, it is also a time that was long expected and might even have been hoped for as a relief from suffering. As my older brother wisely said, and we repeated more than once when we were mourning our mother's death from Alzheimer's disease, "Her death was a loss but not a tragedy."

CHAPTER EIGHT

HOW YOU CAN HELP YOURSELF DURING DIFFICULT TIMES

It makes me feel whole.
—Josef, teen volunteer

Loving someone with dementia, taking care of them, or visiting them can be physically, emotionally, and psychologically hard. It places enormous stress on you and your family. It can leave you feeling exhausted, drained, sad, guilty, overwhelmed, angry, depressed, and mean. It is important—for you, for your family, and for the person with dementia—for you to take care of yourself and keep yourself able to function for yourself and the others in your life. You are of no use to anyone if you can't function well, so one of the most important—and maybe hardest—things you can do is to help yourself.

ADVICE FROM AL:
ACKNOWLEDGE WHAT YOU'RE FEELING

Al says, based on both his experience with his grandmother's decline and his experience as a music therapist,

It's great to have things to do, great to have ways to provide comfort. But because there's nothing you can fix, you can just really *be* there, that's all they want. But it can be overwhelming. That's okay, too. Just recognize it and find ways to deal with it. You will see your parents overwhelmed, but remember that you don't have to take care of them. They are adults, and they are your parents. Feelings will sometimes blow up, but try not to let them overwhelm you. You're all in this together, and you'll get through, whatever it takes.

STAY RESTED

Your habit may have been to stay up on your computer until the early morning hours and then crash for a couple of hours before school, maybe sleeping until the afternoon on weekends, if you could get away with it. But dealing with the stress of loving someone with dementia, even if you may not *feel* stressed, will wear you down physically and emotionally, and it is more important than ever that you try to get enough sleep. Turn off the blue screens earlier; read a boring book for a little while in bed and try to turn the light off at an hour that allows you to get about eight hours of sleep per night. You'll find yourself better able to deal with things and have the energy to do the things you need to do when you've gotten enough rest.

FIND JOY IN DOING THINGS FOR YOURSELF

Although I've talked about how you can find joy and gratification in helping someone you love who has dementia, it is equally essential for you to give yourself time to relax and do things that you enjoy for yourself. If sports are your thing, try to stay on the team or keep up with practice, if your school and family chores schedule allow. See if you can carve out a few hours a week for a run, swim, or hike. Even shooting hoops for an hour after dinner or whenever you can find the time will help you better deal with the things that may burden you. Go to the movies, a ballgame, or an outing with friends, or even just stroll to the mall.

Get out in nature. Studies have shown that spending time in nature, whether it's walking in a park, being at the shore, or hiking in the wilderness, helps restore emotional balance and reduce stress.[1]

FIND PEOPLE WITH WHOM YOU CAN TALK ABOUT WHAT YOU'RE GOING THROUGH

Finding people with whom you can talk honestly and openly about your feelings and what you are going through can be extremely important in helping alleviate the pressure you might feel. Whether with a friend, relative, therapist, teacher, counselor, or even a stranger, it can be a great relief and comfort to be able to speak about your feelings, the person with dementia, what they are going through, and what you are going through.

Participating in a support group for families of people with dementia can also help. You may be able to find a local support group for families of people with dementia through your community, house of worship, Alzheimer's disease association, hospital, or nursing home. While there are many support groups for caregivers or families of people with dementia, there are few for teens who are facing the experience of having someone with dementia in their close circle. If you cannot find one locally, you might consider starting one of your own. Many teens may be experiencing the decline of an older relative but not realize that what they are seeing is a disease and that some of their peers might be experiencing it, too. Finding others who are experiencing something similar can be a great relief and give you a chance to share your thoughts, experiences, and worries with teens like you. Not only that, but by sharing what you are going through, you can also share ideas, ways to help, and things that have worked for you.

Reach out to your guidance counselor, school nurse, or social worker and see if they might be able to connect you with other teens going through the same thing. Call local hospitals or nursing homes and make inquiries through their social work or volunteer departments to see whether they either have such a group or might be able to help you start one. The local chapters of Alzheimer's disease organizations or the local senior center may also be able to help you get started. Participating in a support group with peers who are going through the same feelings you are can offer you coping skills, resources, understanding, and the possibility of new friendships bonded over a shared experience.

LET YOURSELF LAUGH

Laughter has long been thought to have healing powers; Proverbs 17:22, translated as, "A joyful heart is good medicine,"[2] might be the first such reference. "Laughter reduces pain and allows us to tolerate discomfort. Laughter establishes or restores a positive emotional climate and a sense of connection between two people."[3] Scientists have recently been studying whether laughter can even boost the immune system.[4] You can sense for yourself that laughing is a great healer; it is hard to be morose when you are laughing and can even make you feel better when you are feeling ill. Watching a funny movie, video, or TV show, anything that gets you to laugh, is helpful. If you have a friend you can always laugh with, find ways to spend time with them. If you know there's a favorite movie or show that always makes you laugh, watch it—or parts of it—whenever you feel you need a lift. Don't worry or feel guilty if you find humor in the actions or behaviors of the person with dementia; as long as your laughter is not mean, it can be healthy and a relief to laugh about something they did or said.

FINDING UNEXPECTED HUMOR AND SHARING IT

When my mother was in the moderate to late stages of dementia, still able to speak a little but with little substance or continuity, she did occasionally come out with the funniest puns or wordplay. I never knew whether it came from some deep consciousness or some strange connections her brain was still able to make, but it would sometimes send me into fits of laughter.

I remember very clearly how, one day when I was leaving, I said, "Well, I have to go now to fix dinner." Her quick response was, "Why, is it broken?"

It was so wonderful that I burst out laughing, and then she did, too. I still don't know whether she was laughing at having said something funny or just because she was sharing in my laughter.

LET YOUR FRIENDS HELP

If your friends know about your situation, whether they know the person who has dementia or not, they will probably want to show you that they care. Let them. It is one way in which they can help you; they can offer support—a willing and available ear for your feelings and thoughts. One thing you can do is invite them to visit your grandparents with you; having a friend with you can encourage conversation and be a diversion for both you and your grandparent.

FIND BALANCE IN YOUR LIFE

If you live close enough to see your grandparent often and have the willingness and availability to help, whether by running errands, visiting, or assisting with personal care or activities, chances are you will find it exhausting and emotionally draining, especially in later stages of the illness. It is important to find a balance in your life between your required activities (for instance, school, chores, or an after-school job, as well as family and home responsibilities) and the things you do to ensure that you retain some time for yourself and the activities that help you recoup your energy and emotional balance.

MAKE TIME TO DO THINGS YOU ENJOY

Whether it's staying on your tennis team, acting in the school play, or spending time with your friends, continuing to participate in things you enjoy, even while you and your family find yourselves deeply involved in caring for someone with dementia, can be a crucial outlet that allows you to maintain the energy and emotional strength that are so important when caring for someone with dementia. As long as the activity is not a means to hide or distance yourself from the circumstances or your or your family's needs, but rather a space for relief and mental recuperation, finding time for enjoyment is enormously important at this time in your life. If, for example, you are throwing yourself deep into the world of playing video game for hours and days on end to avoid confronting the needs of your family and the sadness or guilt you feel, that is not healthy or useful behavior.

EXERCISE

Exercise helps boost endorphins—those chemicals in the nervous system that stimulate feelings of pleasure. Exercise also helps increase energy levels and keep you healthy during times of stress.

WRITE

Writing about your feelings, experiences, thoughts, and worries can be a way to process and discharge some of those emotions in a nonhurtful, positive, and productive way. Whether you write in longhand in a special journal or notebook, or type on your computer, expressing yourself in words, even if you never expect—or want—anyone to read them, can help you organize your thoughts, review your feelings, and generally get things off your chest. Writing in a journal, especially one that is private, allows you to express thoughts and feelings you know might be hurtful to another person. You can express your anger, feelings of embarrassment or humiliation, jealousy, resentment, or feelings of guilt; you can get them out on paper or set them out electronically, in the safety of a private space. You are entitled to your feelings and thoughts; what you should take care *not* to do is allow anyone who might be hurt by reading your words to have access to them. If you are honest and open with yourself when you write, it is almost inevitable that some of the things you write might be painful should someone else read them; therefore, take care to protect your writing so that only you have access to it and never run the risk of hurting someone about whom you have written.

You may even find that writing about your experience caring for someone with dementia might be something that can find an appreciative audience. Your school newspaper or local community paper or website might value a well-written article about your personal experience, especially if it is written so that it might resonate with someone else.

VOLUNTEER TO VISIT OTHER PEOPLE WITH DEMENTIA

Why would you choose to volunteer your time visiting people with dementia when you already have a family member with the disease? It may seem counterintuitive. One good reason is that it is an excellent way to learn more about the disease and the ways in which you can interact with someone with cognitive decline. If you become a volunteer through a hospital, nursing home, or senior center, you will likely get some orientation and training in how to approach someone with dementia, how to talk with them, what to expect, and how to deal with different situations you may face. Moreover, like every form of volunteerism, it is good for *you*. You will feel good about yourself in doing something valuable and meaningful for someone else.

Some organizations link volunteers with older adults; Sweet Readers, for example, engages young people in art activities with older people with dementia.[5] Many nursing homes and hospitals train teens to visit and assist older people with memory issues. Community and national organizations involved in Alzheimer's disease and dementia care also offer volunteer opportunities to help seniors with memory disorders through visits, activities, and field trips.

JOSEF: IT MAKES ME FEEL WHOLE

Josef, a teen volunteer at a nursing home, feels strongly about his experience working with elders in the memory care unit. Said Josef,

> Some won't remember us when we come back, some will, and they'll get excited to see me. Some days she remembers me perfectly fine, and some days she won't. But she'll get up, and she'll start dancing with me, and it's amazing. You never know what's going to happen when you get to that floor. It can be a lot to handle one day, but it can also be the best time. It helps me connect with people more. It makes me feel whole.

NOTES

YOU ARE NOT ALONE

1. Walter D. Glanze, *The Signet/Mosby Medical Encyclopedia* (New York: C. V. Mosby Company, 1985).
2. Kathleen Fifield, "Dementia vs. Alzheimer's: How to Understand the Difference—and Why It Matters," *AARP*, June 25, 2019, https://www.aarp.org/health/dementia/info-2018/difference-between-dementia-alzheimers.html (accessed January 28, 2020).
3. World Health Organization, "Dementia," September 19, 2019, https://www.whol.int/news-room/fact-sheets/detail/dementia (accessed January 28, 2020).
4. Chelsia Hart, "Quote: Those with Dementia Are Still People," *Alzheimers.net*, November 5, 2013, https://www.alzheimers.net/carey-mulligan-dementia-quote/ (accessed January 28, 2020).

CHAPTER ONE: WHAT IS DEMENTIA?

1. National Institute on Aging, "What Is Dementia? Symptoms, Types, and Diagnosis," https://www.nia.nih.gov/health/what-dementia-symptoms-types-and-diagnosis (accessed January 28, 2020).
2. Alzheimer's Research UK, "Sir Terry Pratchett: A Watershed Moment for Dementia," February 11, 2017, https://www.dementiablog.org/sir-terry-pratchett-a-watershed-moment-for-dementia/ (accessed January 28, 2020).

3. Centers for Disease Control and Prevention, "What Is Dementia?" https://www.cdc.gov/aging/dementia/index.html (accessed January 28, 2020).

4. National Institute on Aging, "What Is Dementia?" http://www.nia .nih.gov/health/what-dementia-symptoms-types-and-diagnosis (accessed January 28, 2020).

5. National Institute on Aging, "Alzheimer's Disease Research Centers," https://www.nia.nih.gov/health/alzheimers-disease-research-centers (accessed January 28, 2020).

6. National Institute on Aging, "Preventing Alzheimer's Disease: What Do We Know?" https://www.nia.nih.gov/health/preventing-alzheimers-dis-ease-what-do-we-know (accessed January 28, 2020).

7. World Health Organization, "Dementia," September 19, 2019, https:// www.who.int/news-room/fact-sheets/detail/dementia (accessed January 28, 2020).

CHAPTER TWO: WHAT DOES DEMENTIA LOOK LIKE?

1. Ger T. Rijkers and Stephen I. Pelton, "The Old Man's Friend," *Pneumonia* 10, no. 8 (July 2018), https://pneumonia.biomedcentral .com/articles/10.1186/s41479-018-0052-7.

CHAPTER THREE: WHAT TO EXPECT

1. Jean Kwok, *Searching for Sylvie Lee* (New York: HarperCollins, 2019).

2. *Merriam-Webster*, "Dysphasia," https://www.merriam-webster.com /dictionary/dysphasia (accessed January 28, 2020).

CHAPTER FOUR: WHAT YOU CAN DO
TO HELP SOMEONE WITH DEMENTIA

1. Arthur Kleinman, *The Soul of Care: The Moral Education of a Husband and a Doctor* (New York: Penguin/Random House, 2019).

1. Amy Tan, *The Bonesetter's Daughter* (New York: Ballantine, 2019).

CHAPTER FIVE: HOW DOES DEMENTIA
AFFECT FAMILY AND FRIENDS?

1. Philip D. Fletcher et al., "Pain and Temperature Processing in Dementia: A Clinical and Neuroanatomical Analysis," *Brain: A Journal of Neurology* 138, no. 11 (November 2015): 3,360–72, https://www.ncbi.nlm.nih.gov /pmc/articles/PMC4620514.

CHAPTER SIX: ACTIVITIES TO SHARE
WITH SOMEONE WITH DEMENTIA

1. Oliver Sacks, "Wired for Sound," *Oprah Magazine*, December 2008, https://www.oprah.com/omagazine/oliver-sacks-finds-the-bond -between-music-and-our-brains/all (accessed January 28, 2020).

CHAPTER SEVEN: FACING DEATH AND
THE RITUALS OF DEATH AND MOURNING

1. Susan L. Mitchell et al., "The Clinical Course of Advanced Dementia," *New England Journal of Medicine* 361 (October 2009): 1,529–38, https://www.nejm.org/doi/full/10.1056/NEJMoa0902234.
2. Catherine Elton, "Redefining Dementia as a Terminal Illness," *Time*, October 14, 2009, http://content.time.com/time/health/article /0,8599,1930278,00.html (accessed January 28, 2020).

CHAPTER EIGHT: HOW YOU CAN
HELP YOURSELF DURING DIFFICULT TIMES

1. Mathew P. White et al., "Spending at Least 120 Minutes a Week in Nature Is Associated with Good Health and Well-Being," *Scientific Reports* 9, no. 7,730 (2019), https://www.nature.com/articles/s41598 -019-44097-3.

2. *New American Standard Bible*, "Proverbs 17:22," https://www.bible
   gateway.com/passage/?search=Proverbs+17%3A22&version=NASB
   (accessed January 28, 2020).
3. Hara Estroff Marano, "Laughter: The Best Medicine," *Psychology Today*,
   April 5, 2005, https://www.psychologytoday.com/us/articles/200504
   /laughter-the-best-medicine (accessed January 28, 2020).
4. Mary Payne Bennett and Cecile Lengatcher, "Humor and Laughter
   May Influence Health IV: Humor and Immune Function," *Evidence-
   Based Complement Alternative Medicine* 6, no. 2 (June 2009): 159–64,
   https://www.ncbi.nlm.nih.gov/pmc/articles/PMC2686627/.
5. Sweet Readers, https://www.sweetreaders.org/.

RESOURCES

BOOKS

Anderson, Jessica Lee. *Trudy*. Minneapolis, MN: Milkweed Editions, 2005.

Chast, Roz. *Can't We Talk about Something More Pleasant?* New York: Bloomsbury, 2014.

Hyde, Margaret, and John Setaro. *When the Brain Dies First*. New York: Franklin Watts, 2000.

Korman, Gordon. *Pop*. New York: Blazer and Bray, 2011.

Low, Lee-Fay. *Live and Laugh with Dementia: The Essential Guide to Maximizing Quality of Life*. East Gosford, New South Wales, Australia: Exisle Publishing, 2014.

Mace, Nancy L., and Peter V. Rabins. *The 36-Hour Day: A Family Guide to Caring for Persons with Alzheimer Disease, Related Dementing Illnesses, and Memory Loss in Later Life*. Baltimore, MD: Johns Hopkins University Press, 1999.

Ros, Hana. *Neurocomic*. Illustrated by Matteo Farinella. London: Nobrow Press, 2014.

Sabat, Steven R. *Alzheimer's Disease and Dementia: What Everyone Needs to Know*. New York: Oxford University Press, 2018.

Shea, Therese. *Dementia: Understanding Brain Diseases and Disorders*. New York: Rosen, 2012.

Simpson, Kathleen. *The Human Brain: Inside Your Body's Control Room*. Washington, DC: National Geographic, 2009.

Snyman, Matthew, and Social Innovation Lab Kent. *The Dementia Diaries: A Novel in Cartoons*. London: Jessica Kingsley, 2016.

Sonnenblick, Jordan. *Curveball: The Year I Lost My Grip*. New York: Scholastic Paperbacks, 2014.

Wayman, Laura. *A Loving Approach to Dementia Care: Making Meaningful Connections with the Person Who Has Alzheimer's Disease or Other Dementia or Memory Loss*, 2nd ed. Baltimore, MD: Johns Hopkins University Press, 2017.

ORGANIZATIONS

Alzheimer's Association
25 North Michigan Avenue, 17th Floor
Chicago, IL 60601
800-272-3900
https://www.alz.org/help-support/resources/kids-teens/for_teens
This link offers information for teens from the Alzheimer's Association, the leading voluntary health organization devoted to Alzheimer's care, support, and research.

Alzheimer's Association Hotline
800-272-3900
This confidential telephone hotline, manned by professional staff, is available 24 hours a day, 365 days a year, to people living with the disease, their families, caregivers, and the public. The hotline offers support, information, and referrals to resources on every aspect of Alzheimer's disease and dementia.

Alzheimer's Disease Research Centers
https://www.nia.nih.gov/health/alzheimers-disease-research-centers
The National Institute on Aging funds Alzheimer's Disease Research Centers (ADRCs) at major medical institutions throughout the United States. Researchers at these centers are working to translate research advances into improved diagnosis and care for people with Alzheimer's disease, as well as working to find a treatment or way to

prevent Alzheimer's and other types of dementia. For patients and families affected by Alzheimer's disease the ADRCs offer help with obtaining diagnosis and medical management; information about the disease, services, and resources; opportunities for volunteers to participate in clinical trials and studies and patient registries; and support groups and other special programs for volunteers and their families.

American Association of Caregiving Youth
6401 Congress Avenue, Suite 200
Boca Raton, FL 33432
561-391-7401
https://www.aacy.org/

A nonprofit organization, the American Association of Caregiving Youth is the only organization in the United States dedicated solely to addressing caregiving youth issues. Their goal is to help every youth caring for chronically ill, injured, elderly, or disabled family members achieve success in school and life; increase awareness; and provide support services for youth caregivers and their families by connecting them with healthcare, education, and community resources.

FILMS

Age-Old Friends (1989) (TV movie)

John, a nursing home resident, spends time with his best buddy, Michael, who's slowly drifting into senility. The movie portrays the fight for independence and dignity in old age.

Alive Inside: A Story of Music and Memory (2014)

A passionate documentary about the power of music to reach the hearts and souls of dementia patients with the help of an iPod. The film follows social worker Dan Cohen as he uses music to "awaken" patients with dementia and Alzheimer's. Bedridden individuals come to life as they hear songs from their youth.

Aurora Borealis (2005)
With Juliette Lewis and Donald Sutherland, this movie is about a troubled young man who struggles to find himself as he deals with his father's decline into dementia.

Away from Her (2007)
Starring Julie Christie, Olivia Dukakis, and Michael Murphy, this movie details how a long-married couple deals with the wife's decline into dementia.

Firefly Dreams (2001) (Japanese, English subtitles)
Naomi, a spoiled teenager from Nagoya, is sent off to the country for the summer to work at her aunt's inn. After being asked to care for an aging relative with Alzheimer's disease, Naomi develops an extraordinary friendship with the older woman that changes her perspective on life.

Glen Campbell: I'll Be Me (2014)
This documentary follows country-music legend Glen Campbell as he struggles with Alzheimer's disease and embarks on a farewell tour.

Iris: A Memoir (2001)
Starring Judi Dench and Kate Winslet, this movie is based on the true story of the lifelong romance between novelist Iris Murdoch and her husband, John Bayley, from their student days through her battle with Alzheimer's disease.

My Name Is Lisa (Shelton Films, YouTube)
https://www.youtube.com/watch?v=ZiRHyzjb5SI
This is a six-and-a-half-minute dramatization of a young teen facing her mother's decline into dementia.

The Notebook (2004)

With Gena Rowlands, Rachel McAdams, and James Garner, this is a romantic story of memory, age, and love.

A Quick Look at Alzheimer's

https://www.agingresearch.org/video/quicklookatalzheimers1/

This series of short, animated films offers an introductory understanding of Alzheimer's disease.

The Savages (2007)

Actress Laura Linney and actor Philip Seymour Hoffman are siblings who must face the realities of familial responsibilities as they begin to care for their ailing father.

Sir Terry Pratchett: Living with Alzheimer's (2009)

https://www.youtube.com/watch?v=KmejLjxFmCQ

In this two-part documentary, the best-selling author of the Discworld series, who died of Alzheimer's disease in March 2015, at age sixty-six, describes his experience of living with dementia.

A Song for Martin (2001) (Swedish, English subtitles)

Swedish composer/conductor Martin and concertmaster Barbara fall in love. After their divorces, they're happily married. While composing an opera, Martin is diagnosed with Alzheimer's disease.

Still Alice (2014)

In this poignant film, Julianne Moore plays a linguistics professor who learns she is experiencing early-onset Alzheimer's disease. She and her family must face her progressive decline.

WEBSITES

Alzheimer's Association
"Facts and Figures"

https://www.alz.org/alzheimers-dementia/facts-figures
National Institute on Aging
"Resources for Children and Teens about Alzheimer's Disease"
https://www.nia.nih.gov/healthresources-children-and-teens-about
    -alzheimers-disease

National Institute on Aging
"What Is Dementia? Symptoms, Types, and Diagnosis"
https://www.nia.nih.gov/healthwhat-dementia-symptoms-types-and
    -diagnosis

SONGS TO SING TOGETHER

If you don't know these songs by heart, they're easily found on the
    internet on such sites as www.genius.com. If you can play an instru-
    ment in accompaniment, that can add an extra level of engage-
    ment, but just singing together is wonderful on its own.
"Amazing Grace"
"America the Beautiful"
"Bicycle Built for Two (Daisy Bell)"
"The Daring Young Man on the Flying Trapeze"
"God Bless America"
"Goodnight, Irene"
"Let It Be"
"My Bonnie Lies Over the Ocean"
"Oh, Give Me a Home"
"Que Sera, Sera (Whatever Will Be, Will Be)"
"Raindrops Keep Falling on My Head"
"Somewhere Over the Rainbow"
"This Land Is Your Land"
"Twinkle, Twinkle, Little Star"
"You Are My Sunshine"

INDEX

ABOUT THE AUTHOR

Jean Rawitt is a former executive in book publishing, marketing, public relations, and fundraising. She trained in geriatrics education at the Hunter/Mount Sinai Geriatrics Education Center and went on to develop volunteer programs for Mount Sinai Hospital in New York City, including one for high school volunteers, to help offset the negative effects of hospitalization on the frail elderly. Rawitt is also author of *Volunteering: Insights and Tips for Teenagers* (Rowman & Littlefield, 2020).